# THE HIGH COST OF HEALING

# THE HIGH COST OF HEALING

*Physicians and the Health Care System*

## J.H.U. Brown, Ph.D.

*Professor*
*University of Houston*
*Adj. Professor Public Health Administration*
*University of Texas Health Science Center*
*Houston, Texas*

1985

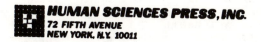

**HUMAN SCIENCES PRESS, INC.**
**72 FIFTH AVENUE**
**NEW YORK, N.Y. 10011**

54287

Copyright © 1985 by Human Sciences Press, Inc.
72 Fifth Avenue, New York, New York 10011

Printed in the United States of America
987654321

**Library of Congress Cataloging in Publication Data**

Brown, J. H. U. (Jack Harold Upton),
    The high cost of healing.

    Bibliography: p.
    Includes index.
    1. Medical care, Cost of—United States.  2. Physi-
cians—United States.  3. Medical care—United States.
I. Title.  [DNLM: 1. Cost Control.  2. Delivery of Health
Care—economics—United States.  3. Ethics, Medical.
4. Physicians.  W 74 B878h]
RA410.53.B76  1985      338.4'33621'0973      84-10823
ISBN 0-89885-222-6

# CONTENTS

# PREFACE

As the cost of the medical system rises steadily and places greater burdens upon the average taxpayer, recriminations are beginning to mount. Each element of the system blames the other for the rising costs and the often poor service. We are a litigative society and as a result the cost of malpractice is increasing and more and more physicians practice defensive medicine regardless of the cost and, to some extent, the welfare of the patient.

This book is an attempt to look at some of the parameters which determine the quality and cost of care, dealing primarily with the physician. There are several distinct steps which led to the physician's disregard of costs, and each will be discussed in turn. Medical education is a tertiary medical care training system and does not deal with cost reduction or cost control. The medical student is trained to use all of the armamentarium of care and to use it lavishly.

When the physician goes into practice much of this learning period is carried forward. Residency and specialty training increase the costs of care. Residents are trained largely in highly circumscribed areas with highly developed technology and do not know the costs of the procedures they order so freely.

The hospital is not as much to blame as the physician. The

hospital writes no orders and carries out no procedures. But the hospital makes a great deal of money from high technology and is not loath to use it and to encourage the physician to use it. This is especially true of the laboratory where vast numbers of unused tests are performed and discarded.

The insurance system and the patient are also to blame, but again under the physician's aegis. The patient demands tertiary care but it is the physician who must assign space and order drugs. The patient and the physician are unconcerned about the costs of care because the insurance companies serve as a middle man to insulate both from the costs/benefit factors.

Finally, medical ethics play an important part in the cost of care. The "right to live" and the "right to die" issues place strains on the costs of care, and the overbearing threat of malpractice requires a different standard of care aimed largely at protection of the physician.

This is the plan of the book. We will discuss first the costs of the system. These have been overemphasized in the news-papers but are still an issue. We will then examine the factors influencing care. The role of the physician, in private practice, in the hospital, and in the technological scene will be considered. In order to reach this point we shall have to discuss the factors of medical education and the way that education molds the future physician.

Finally we will look at the ancillary factors affecting practice, including ethics, insurance, and other such problems.

In each case we will suggest solutions to some of the problems. Many of the solutions may be real answers but may be unobtainable in the context of the political and social environment in which we live. Many of us may live to see the changes. If we are to end up with a health care system which is equitable to all we must make a beginning.

# A BRIEF EXPLANATION

It must be emphasized that this book is not a diatribe against hospitals and physicians. Neither is it an attempt to whitewash the profession. I have many friends among physicians who in the main are dedicated, hardworking, and conscientious individuals. However, in a population of 450,000 persons we are likely to have a mixture of honesty and dishonesty, patience and impatience, much as one would expect in the general population. In addition, each physician is apt to have a family to support, and money becomes an important element in the making of his decisions. All of these factors, operating within one of the largest industries in the world, leads to abuses which will be discussed later. I apologize in advance to those physicians who do not recognize themselves or their behavior in the examples given. The examples are chosen mainly to make a point, to emphasize an aspect of health care and do not reflect on physicians as a whole. However, the entire picture *does* reflect on both physician and hospitals and suggest that reform must come before we reach an impossible-to-resolve conflict between the public, the government, and the health care system.

# Chapter 1

# INTRODUCTION

As we are faced with a cost of medical care which is rising about twice as fast as the cost of living, with a productivity which is decreasing from year to year and with a gradually increasing impersonal approach, the American public is beginning to question the health care system as a whole. In general, the blame is usually placed on several factors:

The increasing costs of technology
The increasing demand for care
The increasing use of tertiary care
The failure to develop a preventive system

Although each of these has its roots in a different part of the system, the laboratory, the hospital, the ancillary care facilities, in the ultimate analysis it is the physician who is to blame.

Although the physicians deny their responsibility (Owens, 1983), it is clear that no patient would be assigned to a hospital, no patient would have expensive tests performed, no patient would be subjected to surgery without the direct order of a physician. Again, as the physician and the system is geared to the treatment of the sick, there is little emphasis upon prevention. In fact, the recent decline in deaths from heart disease and certain cancers can be more easily attributed to the change in personal habits (less smoking, more exercise, better diet) than to any medical intervention. This single example embodies all of the problems of medical care. Most of the increase in life span has come about from factors other than medical care. The short life span of the 1800–1900s was mainly due to the death of children from the common diseases of measles, diphtheria, scarlet fever, etc. The prevention of these diseases by vaccination during the early part of the century made by far the greatest change in mortality to date.

An indication that life style is the fundamental cause of illness rather than the familiar bacteria has been amply demonstrated. Data provided by the DHHS indicates that as women began to smoke the incidence of cancer of the mouth and lung increased rapidly by as much as 84 percent in thirty years. The evidence is also clear that smoking and the drinking of alcohol damages the fetus during pregnancy and that our life style now reflected in woman's behavior has resulted in increased cardiovascular disease, bronchitis, and emphysema among that group. Furthermore, the situation is worsening. More girls are starting to smoke than boys and are apparently smoking more. The situation is abetted by the widespread advertising of cigarettes, the support of women's sports by cigarette companies, and the failure of the physician to point out the problems in strong terms to decrease the effects.

Although we spend large sums of money on the treatment of acute illness, we are neglecting the major illnesses among us. For example, DHHS reports that Alzheimer's disease is now the fourth leading cause of death in the United States. The disease is incurable, occurs only in the elderly, and is essentially untreatable. Alzheimer's disease has been listed as the cause of more than 50 percent of all nursing home admissions and costs about $10 billion per year. Yet we do very little for the elderly, and geriatric medicine is a neglected subject in most medical schools.

Prevention is the neglected portion of the health care system. The physician does not teach prevention and is not to be credited with much effort at prevention because it is not in the doctor's best interests. But prevention is effective. Diphtheria was reduced from 160,000 cases and 10,000 deaths per year in 1920 to 59 cases and four deaths by 1980. Measles caused about 5,000 deaths in 1930 and six in 1978. Polio was represented by 21,000 cases in 1952 and 26 in 1979. In 1960 there were about 500,000 cases of measles and in 1979 there were about 14,000. This did not come about because of the practice of medicine. The major influence was the requirement in all 50 states that children be vaccinated before entering school. The strides in disease eradication can thus be attributed to public health measures and the development of the vaccine rather than to any effort on the part of the health system represented by the hospital and the physician.

We can illustrate the problem with a simple figure (Fig. 1). In general, the simple procedures such as vaccination, diet, and other preventive measures can be supplied to large numbers of people at very low cost. On the other hand, the very complicated procedures, such as open heart surgery, can be supplied to only a very few people at extremely great expense. In addition, the

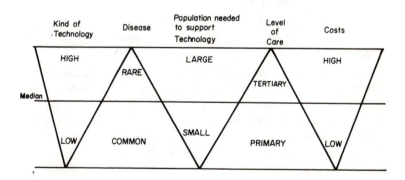

**Figure 1.** The relationship between the availability, costs, and degree of technology, and the number of patients helped in a health care system. (Taken from Brown, *Politics of Health Care*, Cambridge: Ballinger Press, with permission.)

use and cost of technology is proportional to the same factors. The use of vaccinations as opposed to open heart surgery is a low-tech, low-expense venture.

Many of the faults of the system can be attributed to the physician, but he or she is not entirely to blame. We may assign blame to:

The education of the physician
The demands of a hypochondriac population
The competition between hospitals for patients and staffs
The failure of the population to heed most warnings about life styles

In addition to the more obvious reasons for increasing costs of medical care, we must also look at other less well-known but equally potent factors. These include:

Defensive medicine
Failure to obtain coordination in the health care system
Specialization in medicine
Political disputes in medical regulations
The conflict between ethical and economical medical care

In order to examine these influences and determine the solution to the problems we must begin, as does the average physician, in medical school. The medical schools of the country are still 40 years behind the times in terms of the future directions of medicine. Emphasis has been placed upon medical technology and its use in tertiary medical care. Few medical schools teach courses in such necessary topics as office management, economics of medical care, ambulatory care, and the elements of preventive medicine. Concentration is devoted to the basic medical sciences and to the more esoteric diseases which occur in the teaching hospital but which occur in real life in about 1 percent of the patients. Several recent studies (Zeleznick, 1983) have pointed out that students do equally well in medical school regardless of prior training. In fact, some educators have suggested that medical students would probably be better physicians if they came from a social science rather than a hard science background. While it is true that the physician needs physiology, pathology, anatomy, etc. for the practice of medicine, it is doubtful if a physician in private practice ever again considers the role of glucose-6-phosphatase in his or her practice.

Today the average medical student progresses from basic to clinical sciences within the 4-year span. Under most circumstances, the clinical areas are divided into carefully segregated and nonoverlapping specialties. The student sees the ob/gyn patient today and the cardiac patient tomorrow. He or she rarely sees the average patient with multiple problems, many of which may be minor. During this entire period the student is taught by specialists and encouraged to be a specialist. Is there any wonder that 90 percent of all medical students enter a specialty (JAMA, 1981)? No one bothers to tell the prospective doctor that 85 percent of patients will be ambulatory with about 15 common diseases including aches and pains, colds, intestinal disorders, and a variety of other equally mundane problems, or that adrenal hyperplasia, about which the doctor studied in medical school, is likely to occur once in a lifetime.

Yet all of the people must be served regardless of the problem. The medical problem may be minor to the physician but it is major to the suffering patient. Although there has been lip service to the practice of family medicine and the general practitioner, the actual fact is that both family practice and general physicians are seeing a decrease in income and in patient load (Owens, 1983). A part of this is due to the emphasis given the specialist by the profession, so the patient becomes convinced that the specialist is the only road to wellness.

## THE AMERICAN HEALTH CARE SYSTEM

We are told with increasing frequency and with doubtful assurance that the United States has the finest health care system in the world. It is true that we spend more per capita on health care than any other nation, but money does not always assure quality. At the moment the United States ranks about nineteenth in the rate of infant mortality. While it is true that many of the nations with low rates have nothing like the polyglot mixture of population which we enjoy, it is also true that many of those nations spend one quarter or less of the amount per person we do on health care. It should be apparent that with the large expenditures we should be able to do better.

We have many areas of the country with no physicians and other areas with almost none. By far the largest percentage of all doctors live in the big cities and cannot be encouraged to move to rural areas. Other countries have made a greater success in this regard by fiat, inducement, or medical education.

At the moment we are not the longest lifed nation on earth. Japanese men and women live longer than Americans, and Iceland, Sweden, Norway, and the Netherlands all have longer life spans than we enjoy.

It can be cited with some justification that in the time of Moses a person was said to live threescore years and ten. After 6,000 years of medicine that expectancy has increased to about threescore years and eighteen. We have defeated the diseases which can be treated with prevention, but we have made few inroads on the chronic diseases of arthritis, cancer, and heart disease. The one improvement in life statistics has been the reduction in deaths by heart attacks and almost all of the reduction is credited to improvement in life style, such as reduction of smoking, better diet, and exercise.

From another viewpoint, it could be argued that the amounts spent on medical care have actually decreased the quality of care rendered in specific instances. There appears to be no question that many more people are subjected to hysterectomies, to kidney dialysis, and to heart bypass surgery than need the procedures. Many people suffer more in the hospital from iatrogenic disease than they do from the disease for which they entered the institution. The population in general takes more drugs, sees more doctors, and has more procedures than are necessary.

These few facts point out that the health care system in the United States has many faults. On the other hand, it does provide a high standard of care albeit at high cost, and it probably provides what the American people want. The question is whether what the people want is good for them.

## The High Costs of Care

Each year the Federal government publishes masses of statistics on the health care system. The Health Care Financing Administration (HCFA) analyzes the data and summarizes much of the material. From these sources we can draw a picture of the health care system and its costs.

In 1982 we spent $287 billion on health care. This enormous amount totaled almost 10 percent of the GNP or, in simpler terms, about $1,225 per person or almost $4,000 per family. About 32 percent of this sum was paid by the consumer in direct costs and the rest was paid by insurance, governmental sources, and other secondary sources. Hospitals collected about 40 percent of the total while the physicians received about 20 percent. Overall, some 43 percent of the bill was paid by taxes from federal, state, or local venues. The disparity of the distribution becomes obvious when we consider that of the $287 billion, some $21 billion was spent on drugs but only $7 billion on public health; some $7 billion was spent on health facility construction but less than $1 billion on prevention of disease.

Current data suggests that there are about 280 physicians for every 100,000 people in New York, an increase from 239/100,000 only 10 years ago. During the same period the number of gastroenterologists has increased 43 percent, pediatricians 24 percent, and orthopedists 17 percent, while general practitioners have decreased 28 percent. It is difficult to argue that the number of ulcers in New York has increased 43 percent or the population has increased 24 percent in a 10-year period. When we consider that an average of about one physician per 1,000 people is sufficient to operate an HMO and provide more than adequate medical services, there is little wonder that physicians in New York are finding it difficult to establish practice, obtain hospital affiliations, and compete with established physicians who may resent their intrusion into an already overcrowded area.

The distribution of health care varies widely. In New York City there are about 280 physicians/100,000 people, while in some areas of Texas there are entire counties with no physicians. The state of Massachusetts spent about $935 per person on health care for its citizens while South Carolina spent $521. Hospitals received $490/person in Massachusetts but $197 in Idaho. Of greater concern is the ever-escalating cost of care. At the moment the cost of care is increasing about twice the rate of the GNP (12 percent vs. 5 percent). The present predictions are that health care will cost $756 billion in 1990, about 13 percent of the GNP or $3,000 per person, $12,000 per family. One reason for the increase is that both the supply of lawyers and the supply of physicians is increasing at about three times the rate of increase of the population as a whole. Last year there were about 600 million ambulatory visits by patients to the health care system. About 11 percent of the entire population (23 million) visited some form of outpatient department or emergency room. The role of the emergency room has been called into question because fewer than 14 percent of those visiting emergency clinics had a life-threatening emergency.

The number of visits can be correlated with the advent of medical insurance. About 88 percent of the population is covered by medical insurance. Of this large group almost 40 percent pay no premiums, another 38 percent pay some but not all of the premiums, and the remainder pay their own premiums. The average family pays about $470 per year out of pocket for total medical care. This is insignificant when we consider that last year the average hospital bill was $2,851 and the average daily charge for a hospital bed was $165.

These statistics were derived from Freeland (1983), Chyba (1983), Dicker (1983), Levit (1982), and Gibson (1982), in order to present a general picture of the present situation.

The Health Care Financing Review has presented a variety of facts regarding the use of the health care system. Most of the data are discouraging. For example, there has been a 35 percent increase in hospital populations during a period when the population as a whole increased only 10 percent; surgery increased 53 percent during the same period. Cardiovascular surgery also increased 150 percent for persons over sixty-five as compared to those under that age. Although some of the increase can be attributed to increase in the number of older persons compared to the rest of the population, or to improvements in techniques which permitted a greater number to be operated on with less risk, the discrepancy is too large to be explained by the demographic factors (Lubitz, 1982) and suggests response to payment by the government, increase in physician population, and other economic factors.

## WHY HEALTH CARE COSTS RISE

Feldstein (1977) has suggested that the rise in health care costs can be divided into two areas: the "how" medical costs rise and the "why" medical costs rise. The two areas are clearly distinguishable from each other. Under "How" can be lumped the general rise of costs in general, the growth of the population, the growth in demand, the increase in technology and services provided, and the overinflation of medical care costs. The "Why" includes such topics as birth and death rates, fiscal policies of the government, factors which effect the supply and demand for medical care including insurance payments, fee for service, technology, shifts in the sex-age ratios of the population, increases in income, availability of services, etc. Feldstein's argument is a sound one except that it does not approach the real facts. We must explain not the increase in costs which occur for the usual demographic reasons, which can be estimated with great precision, but rather those increases which are twice the rate of growth of the GNP and to which no definite reasons can be attached. Of even greater importance is the fact that the increase in cost above the GNP cannot be correlated with improvement in health status or in the cure of disease.

Lewis Thomas, in *Lives of a Cell*, has pointed out that we live in an era of what he calls "half-technology" where high tech is used primarily for palliation rather than prevention or cure. If we fail to cure a disease with medicine, it must be apparent that the cost benefit of the treatment is very low and if we prolong life at the expense of life style or well-being, we could argue that the cost benefit may be negative rather than positive. In the ultimate we must look to "more bang for the bucks."

As the costs of health care rise above 10 percent of the GNP and the threats to the Social Security system increase, we become more and more aware of the problems which face us now and in the immediate future. While there is no limit to be set on the cost of health care, i.e., there is no fiscal reason why we should not pay 20 percent of the GNP for health if we so desire, practically, resistance has arisen, in resistance to taxes, and in the demand for reform that began where the cost of health care reached 8 percent of the GNP. (And this cost is steadily increasing.) There is a generally uncomfortable feeling that the quantity of care is in excess of need. The United States now spends more on health care as a percentage of the GNP than any other country including such cradle-to-the-grave systems as that in Sweden. Yet as we have remarked above, our system does not produce a markedly better care.

The overutilization of services in the United States is apparent when costs are compared to those of another well-developed country—France (NCHS, 1983). The cost of an average stay in the hospital in France is about one-half that of the cost in the United States. The United States uses about twice as many personnel to deliver the same services. The discrepancy becomes greater when it is realized that in France 99 percent of the population is covered by compulsory health insurance and are therefore freer to use the system.

The impact of high costs is making inroads into the services which the states will provide under Medicare. California has dropped from its rolls 121 hospitals which refused to give discounts to Medicare patients; South Carolina has limited hospital days to 12 per year, and Missouri has limited doctors visits to two per month. Other states are requiring the patient to pay for part of services, such as prescription drugs, while others are requiring the patient be removed from nursing homes when home care can be provided.

## BIG BUSINESS AND THE HEALTH CARE SYSTEM

Any part of the economy which spends $287 billion in a single year is big business. The health care industry employs millions of workers, hundreds of thousands of doctors, has hundreds of billions invested in buildings and equipment, and purchases billions of dollars of supplies each year. The health care payroll is about 65 percent of the total amount expended in health care and represents an enormous segment of the total economy.

The presence of a large relatively homogenous market has attracted a variety of industrial giants. Drugs alone comprise a $25 billion market. Because the system is a not-for-profit, retrospective payment system where costs are billed after the patient has been treated, incentives exist for large profits in the industrial sector. There are about 10,000 formulations of drugs on the market including 1,200 specific drugs in 4,000 forms of administration. Seventy-five percent of all patients receive drugs on visits to the physician and 85 percent of these drugs are prescription. Furthermore, 35 percent of those receiving drugs get two prescriptions and an additional 23 percent get three prescriptions per visit (Cypress, 1982). Most of the drugs (88 percent) were proprietary rather than generic due primarily to the good work of retail people and the advertising media.

The for-profit hospital chains, which are expanding rapidly, now claim about $16 billion of the health care budget with returns on their investment of perhaps 10 percent. The very idea that profit-making entities can come into the health care field and not only compete with the present system but make money, suggests that the system is fat and can easily be trimmed to more reasonable proportions. Booming technology has also created a big business. The implantation of 50,000 pacemakers at about $500 each (not counting surgical costs), the rapid influx of CAT and PET scanners, and now NMR and other diagnostic tools with high price tags (up to $1 million each) have created a business in technology solely for the medical field and such companies as Technicon deal only with medical problems.

Even relatively low-cost items such as infant monitoring and prenatal monitoring equipment at about $15,000 per unit are big business because of the enormous volume.

The big business attracts ancillary groups. Unions are actively recruiting members in the hospital staffs, lawyers specialize in malpractice suits, there are makers of uniforms and packers of special diets. Each arises because of the possibility of profit and each contributes to the rise in costs.

The physician and the hospital are also to blame. Much

equipment is purchased on the basis of smart advertising. The hospital laboratory is a lucrative source of income for the hospital and the use of high tech equipment to increase the number of tests performed per unit of time is good business for the hospital if not for the patient.

We will return again to these problems in the pages ahead as we examine the contribution of the physician to the problems and their solutions.

The profits which can be made from a clinical laboratory have attracted the large corporations. Many clinical labs are now operated as for-profit organizations with large returns to the investors. The take-over of clinical labs results in increased prices, increased use of tests, and increased lobbying for concessions on standards. Bailey (1977) found that clinical labs are in fierce competition and as a result are often willing to make concessions to the physician in discounts for large numbers of tests, etc. This encourages the physician to use more tests.

The country has in one sense determined the treatment for disease. The response of Congress to fears of the populace has resulted in large appropriations for the dread diseases. However, the fear of the country has not been in step with the incidence of disease. We now tremble at the word AIDS (Acquired Immune Deficiency Syndrome) yet only 6,500 people have ever contracted the disease. Almost this many are injured each week in highway accidents. Mushkin (1979) pointed out that in 1978 the National Cancer Institute spent about $762 million for a disease causing 366 deaths per 100,000 people and an average of 4.6 work days lost per person. The National Heart and Lung Institute spent $370 million for 804 of each 100,000 deaths and 55 days lost and the National Institute of Arthritic and Metabolic Disease spent $80 million for 109 deaths/100,000 and 77 days lost. It is obvious that the fear of a disease rather than its prevalence or actual risk is the determining factor for governmental action.

We have squandered resources in medicine. One can argue that there is an ethical reason for the use of high technology and, in fact, this is the argument so often applied. However, one can also reason that the expenditure of 1 percent of our resources for health care on 0.25 percent of the population who must have renal dialysis is an unwarranted segregation of resources. The same argument could be applied to the 200,000 who obtain a cardiac bypass each year at a cost of about $3 billion in direct costs, where 0.04 percent of the patients receive 1 percent of the financial benefits of treatment. Similar arguments could be made about heart and liver transplants. When one considers that we spend 0.5 percent of our medical dollars on prevention which might eliminate some of the diseases listed above, the argument can be made that our priorities should be adjusted (Evans, 1983).

In addition, much technology is poorly used. The thermograph a few years ago was the diagnostic method of choice for the detection of breast cancer. Recent data (Libshitz, 1978) suggest that thermography may be only 50 percent effective and has a high number of false positives which can be almost as disturbing and dangerous as false negatives.

What is the end result? The data suggest that many procedures are attempted on the basis of word-of-mouth reports. Controlled clinical trials may prove the results to be by no means as effective as the first impression. An analysis of some 100 studies of effectiveness of cardiac bypass surgery revealed that only four had sufficient case number and controls to be valid studies and most of these were negative in outcome. Secondly, many studies designed to demonstrate the effectiveness of a procedure have no method of determining the real goal of medicine, the final outcome. We tend to measure effectiveness in terms of process evaluation which is only whether the procedure works, not whether the patient is actually benefited or needed the procedure in the first place. (See *Science* 198:677 et seq. 1977).

Two other points should be mentioned. In the first place, the success of medicine is in some doubt. In 1900 there were about 1,650 deaths per 100,000 of which almost 600 were due to infectious disease. Prevention and antibiotics changed the picture so that in 1970 deaths had decreased to 940/100,000 of which 37 were due to infectious disease. Improvement in the treatment of noninfectious disease has not been remarkable. In 70 years we have reduced the number of deaths by about 100/100,000 with the expenditure of hundreds of billions of dollars in medical costs.

The record on improvement of health by medicine does not speak well for medical care. Medical care ranks fifth behind diet, environment, genetics, and life style in ability to change health patterns.

## The Nursing Home

The elderly in the United States will shortly approach 12 percent of the total population. Some 20 percent of these will live part or full time in a nursing home. The costs of nursing homes have multiplied five times within a 10-year period while the number of beds has only doubled. In addition, nursing homes are rife with problems. Only about 25 percent are in compliance with Medicare. It has been estimated that more than 30 percent of all patients in nursing homes are receiving Medicare services that exceed their need. In other words, such patients could be accommodated at home or in domiciliary facilities. On the other hand, it has been estimated that some 82 million bed days in hospitals could be downgraded to nursing home or home care at a potential savings of more than $10 billion.

Nursing home care will cost about $23 billion in 1981 (Freeland, 1980). It has been suggested by Callahan (HCFA, 1980) that these charges could be reduced if families would take some responsibility for disabled elders. There is little question that this procedure would be cost effective especially when the poor quality of care in most nursing homes is taken into account.

## Physician Costs

Productivity in the long run is centered in the physician. It is the physician who makes the diagnosis, suggests the treatment, assigns the hospital or nursing home, determines the time and cost of treatment and collects the fees.

Control of physician behavior would make substantial differences in the cost of care. For these reasons, considerable attention has been paid to regulation of physician costs through PSRO and UR which are attempts to regulate overusage. The physician costs to the medical care system take several forms, each of which must be controlled separately.

There are numbers of cases of fraud in Medicare from overcharges, overbilling, and similar fraudulent practices. There are many individuals who believe that a major cost of low productivity on the part of the physician is due to overtreating the patient. Finally, there are cases of mismanagement which add the cost of iatrogenic disease to the cost of illness. This is not the place to discuss outright fraud. The law courts and federal investigative bodies must handle that problem. The charge that some physicians run Medicaid mills is less easy to deny.

# Chapter 2

# WHERE IT ALL BEGAN

## THE COST OF A MEDICAL EDUCATION

We may have the best system of medical education in the world. We most certainly have the costliest. Most medical schools claim that the costs of training a physician exceed $100,000 for the 4-year period. In most medical schools the student pays a fraction of this cost and even in the school with the highest tuition he pays less than 40 percent. The taxpayer pays most of the rest. The entering medical student is faced with 4 years of medical school, probably a year of internship (variable), and then a residency. Some 8 years must elapse before the young person can enter the practice of medicine. During that time he or she receives a varied and perhaps not very suitable training.

The potential medical student comes to medical school with a background in the hard sciences. Most medical schools carefully list physics, chemistry, mathematics, and a great deal of biology as prerequisites for admission. This forces the premedical student into a mold of high tech, high intensity classes with forceful competition from fellow students. All of this despite clear evidence that the college major makes very little difference in the quality of physician turned out (Zeleznicki, 1983). Students majoring in sociology, psychology, or arts seem to do as well as other students if they take the very minimum of required courses and do well on the MCAT (Medical College Aptitude Test). In the experience of this author some of the best medical students have been engineers who have taken a course in biochemistry, a course in physiology, and a course in genetics and nothing else except the straight engineering curriculum.

The method we have used in the past to select medical students has been an indictment of the profession. We have attempted to select on the basis of rigidity of thought, highly directional motivation, and good grades. We have given little thought to the fact that the successful student is often a success in cut-throat competition with fellow students, one who has argued for every point in each course taken, and one who has developed little insight into human nature or personality. More often than not, successful candidates have applied themselves to the required courses in science, have let all other courses slide, paid little attention to fellow students except for the competition, and have become "grinds." Are these the type of students we want to train to administer to the ill patient? It might be better to require a course in sociology, a course in psychology, and a course in economics before considering the science courses.

Finally, one could question the usefulness of (any) courses now taught in the premedical curriculum. Obviously the student should be given a feeling for biology including genetics, an understanding of physics and a little chemistry. I have seen little evidence that the medical student uses math before, during, or after medical school. In fact, most medical students do not have enough understanding of math to design a controlled experiment (MacLachlan, 1976). In the determination of a cardiac output, dye is injected and the technician is required to integrate the area under a curve to determine the volume of blood ejected by the heart in a given time. I have seen almost no medical student who could perform such a simple task although all of them had math as a required subject. The engineering student who enters medical school has been required to apply math and as a result is capable of using it.

The clinical medical curriculum can be examined with equal

care. There is no possibility that we want to return to the days of Pre-Flexner and teach a hands-on, learn-by-practice type of medicine, or that medicine should not have a firm basic foundation. However, there is some question as to the content or extent of courses taught in medical school. Too often medical school teachers were employed first as researchers and second as teachers. They are required to spend about 40 percent of their time in research and their promotion and success in medicine is governed by the papers they produce and the respect of their colleagues which is based solely on research accomplishment.

As a result, teaching suffers. Often the courses are split into many sections, each taught by a professor, with little or no integration and coordination. The topics are often selected to suit the research interest of the teacher and as a result some topics tend to be emphasized over others, not on the basis of use to the potential physician but because the topic is of interest to the teacher.

Politics becomes a major determinant of the curriculum. The curriculum committee hears from department chairpersons, all of whom believe firmly that they require a full year to train any medical student. The curriculum is carved up on the basis of influence, not on the need of the student. One classic example: we have perhaps twice as many surgeons as we can possibly use in this country (this will be discussed more fully later in the book). Yet a large part of the medical curriculum is devoted to the surgeons. It would appear to be more realistic to say we need primary physicians so one-half or more of the curriculum will be devoted to primary medicine and the other areas will be slighted. On this basis only one or two students would be permitted to take anesthesiology or surgery, or ob/gyn. Although we may never arrive at the situation where departments are eliminated in medical schools, we should certainly consider the balance between departments and the need for the students they train. The percentage of time devoted to that section of the curriculum could be decreased to nothing or almost nothing and the student could be channelled into courses of more pertinence to future practice. Unfortunately, this is unlikely to happen. The surgeons are a politically powerful group in medicine and are unlikely to stand still for decimation of their ranks although the American

College of Surgeons has proposed to limit the number of residencies because the number of surgeons has far outstripped the need.

On the other hand, we have not provided training in areas in which physicians are needed. We discuss the training of primary or family physicians *ad nauseum,* but we have not increased the number appreciably. In fact, surgeons far outnumber primary care physicians in this country. We need more surgeons than primary physicians in no place other than the battlefield.

An interesting study by Ginzburg (1980) suggests that the students in medical schools recognize that they are not receiving the proper training. Most students queried about their goals and training expressed the feeling that they were being trained in specialty tertiary care when the main need was primary care. The bias of instructors and the curriculum forced them into specialties, they believed. If true, this is real indictment of medical training and the aims of medical schools.

## THE RESIDENCY

A student who has graduated from medical school may require further training. In earlier times the student who graduated was eligible to go into practice immediately and many did so. A little later the internship was devised to provide a year of experience beyond the M.D. degree to permit the student to obtain skills not learned in medical school. As medicine became divided into specialties, the student began to take residencies in highly specialized areas and to spend up to 7 years (in neurosurgery) in training before he or she began to practice. The system has been overblown for many years.

At the moment about 85 percent of all graduating medical students take a residency. Their selection is without regard to need for the specialty or to the distribution of physicians. More than 20 percent of all residencies are in surgery although we are surfeited with surgeons in the United States. Because of the surplus of physicians and the demands of some highly specialized areas, the residency has become narrower and narrower. There are now surgeons who are orthopedists doing only back surgery or knee surgery or hip replacement. There are neurosurgeons who do only spinal cord or only head operations.

The specialty provides several advantages to the physician. Owens (1983) has said that the specialist makes about 35 percent more net income than does the general practitioner or the practitioner in family practice. The surgeon makes about three times as much for an equal amount of time as does the internist. It is obvious that much of the residency mystique is based on the dollar. In addition, there is the prestige of being a member of a specialty board and there is a restriction on the breadth of knowledge required.

There is no question that we do not need the specialists we have and whom we are turning out at the rate of 30,000 per year. Great Britain and most other countries of the world seem to maintain an equal standard of care with strict regulation on the number of residencies. In England, about 40 percent or less of the physicians have any kind of specialist certification and most of these are in hospitals as pathologists, radiologists, or house surgeons.

The danger of a highly specialized medical profession has been recognized. Congress has passed laws requiring medical schools to obtain certification from potential doctors that they will enter family practice or general practice. The program has not been a success. Wechler (1978) found that although medical students signed statements that they would enter family practice, in actuality, many did not and, in fact, entered residencies related to family practice such as pediatric cardiology.

The number of residencies far exceeds the number of students available. Every hospital which aspires to become known outside the immediate areas has a residency program. Theoretically, such a program upgrades the staff and improves quality of care. As a result of the excess positions there is heavy competition for students. The choice residencies in the better centers fill rapidly, but the poorer students are avidly sought after by the lesser known training centers. Such a negative competition, where the student is sought because there is a vacancy rather than because the student is highly competent, tends to encourage more specialization and discourage general practice.

The vacant residency programs, and there are many, have

resorted to other means to fill quotas. One of the most successful from the standpoint of warm bodies is the foreign medical graduate. Some of the smaller hospitals are staffed virtually 100 percent with foreign medical graduates, many of whom are poorly trained and many of whom speak limited English. There have been major complaints of lack of communications between such residents and the patients they treat. Another result of such residency programs has been the great increase in the number of for-profit medical schools in Mexico, the Caribbean, and in a few other locations. Williams (1976) pointed out that the quality of care by many foreign graduates is not equivalent to that given by american medical school graduates.

In some respects the selfish motives of the physicians and the hospitals conflict here. The hospitals have established the practice of hiring foreign medical graduates (FMGs) for in-hospital services and in emergency rooms. There are large numbers working in these areas despite the evidence that some 66 percent are unable to pass the examination for board certification (Neskaukas, 1977). Physicians have objected to the use of foreign medical graduates on two grounds: the poor training and the usurpation of positions which could be occupied by better trained and presumably higher paid American trained graduates. The hospitals, on the other hand, obtain a relatively inexpensive pair of hands with some training.

Last year there were 61,000 residents on duty in 4,500 different programs embracing more than 50 specialties. Of these residencies, 15 percent were in surgery. And 15,000 of the residents were graduates of foreign medical schools. Polares (1978) found there were more neurosurgeons in Massachusetts, with a population of 1 million, than in England, with a population of 50 million. Most were poorly trained because of lack of opportunity to do surgery (Wren, 1975).

It must be emphasized that the entire medical care system is oriented to the residency program. The medical schools pay lip service to family practice or the general practice of medicine but little is actually done about it. The faculty of medical schools are all specialists—they were employed because they *were* specialists—and they have little interest outside their speciality. The student is trained in an environment of tertiary care in which the patient is shunted from specialist to specialist. There is little incentive to learn otherwise. On graduating the student is forcibly enrolled in a residency program where every effort is made to show the advantages of specialization. Surgeons train surgeons and it is unlikely that surgeons will stop such training even when the supply of surgeons exceeds demand as it now does.

Some few areas of the country have become concerned about the lack of family physicians and have initiated programs to correct the deficit. Spencer (1983) found that when a regional education program was devised to retain physicians in family practice, the trend still could not be totally reversed. Most of the students still went to large cities with tertiary medical care facilities like those in which they had been trained. A few went to the middle-sized cities with good facilities and almost none went to rural areas where they were badly needed. Our approach has not yet been successful.

Ginzburg (1981) has pointed out that specialization leads to more specialization and higher costs for medical care. This results in competition for beds in hospitals and higher construction costs, and the entire apparatus may result in a decrease in the quality of care.

Other effects arise from the oversupply. The possibilities of cheaper medical care diminish with the increase in physician supply. We will document the costs increase later, but it is pertinent to point out here that other educational programs suffer with the increasing specialization. Several health care work areas and the Congress of the United States have been interested in ancillary personnel who could replace the physicians in many of their tasks. The group is known as Nurse Practitioners (NP), physicians assistants (PA), and similar titles. About 15 years ago there was a definite swing to training of such individuals who could perform many tasks in the medical areas in a cheaper and perhaps more efficient manner than the physician. With the increase in the number of physicians and the competition which is arising, there has been a concerted movement in the medical societies to suppress such training in favor of the physician performing the tasks even though these may be more menial than those demanded in the usual practice. For example, a family birth control clinic in a large city was recently closed at the instigation of the local medical society, not because it was performing poorly but because it was run solely by nurses. Fay Abdellah (1982) has indicated some of these problems in an excellent article.

We have remarked on the British system, which appears to be able to restrict the residencies. In 1979 McLachlin reported that England had about 49,000 MDs of whom 27,000 were in private practice as *primary care physicians,* with an additional 3,500 in community medicine. This represents a much lower percentage of students in specialty areas but also a much lower physician/patient ratio.

There is still another area of high costs to the medical system from residency training. The resident is expensive to train and expensive to maintain. It has been estimated that the average medical school will spend about 60 percent more per patient than on the comparable wards where only patient care is given. In addition, in order to attract residents, high technology must now be available. Most medical students are accustomed to use the CAT scanner and the SMA-12 and any hospital which would attract residents must also have such equipment. A few years ago, when residents were given room and board and $100 a month, the hospital probably made money on them from the standpoint of the medical care provided, the staffing of emergency wards, etc. Nowadays, with the residency salary reaching $30,000, such is not the case. In addition to the higher basic costs, the resident costs the hospital more. There is ample documentation that the resident orders more tests, spends more staff time, has greater service demands than the practitioner with more experience. Questions could be raised, and have been raised about whether the resident is taught to substitute technology for common sense and accuracy of diagnosis (Dixon, 1974; Eisenberg, 1978; Applegate, 1983; Martz, 1978; and Schroeder, 1977). The evidence is clearly presented by Schroeder (1977), who found that for equivalent diseases and outcomes, the community hospital used many fewer tests than did a nearby teaching hospital.

In addition to the costs of residencies there is a rising tide of complaints. Patients complain that residents exhibit poor relationships with their patients, that the social values are not considered, and that residents treat the patients as a part of the apparatus.

There have been suggestions to alter the situation. The diversion of medical students from residencies to general practice ^ has been tried with little apparent success. We have already mentioned that the number of GPs, their income, and the number of patients they see is declining. This reflects a situation brought about by a feeling of physicians themselves that specialist care is better care. With a third party payment system where the patient does not bear the brunt of expenses, it is easier and makes the patient feel safer to demand a specialist. This alone will perpetuate the system.

It is possible to set stricter requirements on training and thus limit the number of available residents where competition would again permit only the best to enter the system. The number of residencies could easily be set at the need rather than the demand and strict examinations could limit the number entering the specialty. Recertification such as that attempted by the American College of Family Practice could eliminate the poorer performers over a period of time. The stigma of second class medicine which is often attached to the family practice residency should be removed. Surgeons should not be allowed to have practices but should be employees of a hospital where no direct conflict of interest would enter into the decision to operate (Crile, 1983). Some related factors are shown in Table 1.

The implementation of these provisions (which is unlikely) would not eliminate the major problem—how to force the re-

**Table 1    The Factors Which Determine the Number of Physicians in the Health Care System, Which Also Indirectly Determines the Cost and Quantity of Medical Care**

| Supply | Demand |
| --- | --- |
| Medical School Enrollment | Population Increases |
| Number of FMGs | Fees or Reimbursements |
| Death or Retirement of Physicians | Specialization |

distribution of physicians to areas where they are not now located. Canada has provided a generous bonus system to encourage physician relocation in the far North. We may be forced to return to the system used by the University of North Carolina some years ago where students were required to practice in remote areas for a period of time following graduation if they received funds from the state. Since most medical schools have medical education subsidized by taxation, it would be relatively simple to require all students to perform service after graduation or pay the total costs of the medical education from their own pockets. The costs of education could be reduced for a number of years of service rendered and could be essentially free for a long enough period. It can be argued that this is servitude. That is pure nonsense. In a real sense, the servitude is imposed on those who must pay taxes to bear the exorbitant costs of medical care training for a physician who will average about $90,000 a year in net income for the remaining 40–50 years of life. If we were terribly short of physicians and if residencies were not filled, one might consider incentives. At the moment and for the foreseeable future we need negative incentives.

The actual closure of some medical schools and restriction of enrollment of others would be in the best interests of the country. Texas has six medical schools, training 1,200 doctors per year. A case could be made for training this many physicians if the state population and the death or retirement of physicians resulted in an increase of 1,000 in population for each added physician. Since it is unlikely that the state will increase by 1,200,000 people per year even in a rapidly expanding population boom, we are training too many doctors. Part of the reason is politics. At least one governor wanted a medical school in his area despite the lack of clinical facilities. Another wanted a medical school in a large university to compete with medical schools in the other state university system. Such profligate disregard for public expenditures has resulted in a high cost system which is self-perpetuating. The high costs continue because politicians and the general public are unaware of medical economics. Although this will be brought up again later it should be mentioned that an increase in doctors does not result in competition and lower prices and better care. Instead it results in higher prices as each physician maintains a personal income in the face of a decreasing workload by increasing fees, and it results in poorer care because as physicians, especially surgeons, see fewer patients, the skills are not as well maintained and more mistakes are made.

It is difficult to close a medical school. There has been a tremendous investment in buildings, people, and apparatus. Most medical schools are multistory enormous edifices with little demonstrated need for the entire facility. They expand relentlessly. The faculty needs research space, patients must be brought in and studied, and the student must be provided with amenities. Every medical school prides itself upon the range and depth of research conducted on the premises. No one questions the fact that this research often accomplishes little. Because the faculty are oriented by specialty training to the sick rather than the well, the research emphasis is the cure of the sick. This is "half-medicine" and does not reflect the thrust of prevention. We can reiterate one point in this regard. The reduction in heart disease and the slight declines in some forms of cancer may be attributed not to the medical school research but to the change in life styles of the population. There is little evidence that the billions spent have provided great improvement in outcomes.

In summary, we need to rethink our objective in medical education and to outline a different pathway for the medical student to follow. We need to change the residency system to one of need rather than one of preference and we need to determine how many physicians can provide necessary care and limit the expansion of the system to that number. Finally, we need to provide incentive for general practice, for practice in rural areas of need, and we need to decrease our reliance on technology in favor of more common sense and good practice.

Dr. David Rogers of the Robert W. Johnson Foundation has proposed several advances in the education of medical students (Knowles, 1977). The best suggestion is that all students be taken out of the hospital and trained in outpatient or ambulatory care rather than tertiary care. Secondly, he has proposed that two classes of MD be recognized at the outset—the generalist and the specialist. It is not easy to see how we can force students into two pathways unless we have tests which can clearly distinguish between them. In English medical schools the distinction is clear.

About 80 percent of all students go into general practice and only a few become specialists (MacLachan, 1979).

Finally, a recent article in the *New England Journal of Medicine* (Eichna, 1983) proposed that we look again at the entire medical curriculum. The last year should be completely restructured from tertiary care. Faculty should be required to teach by lesson plan in specific subjects rather than in areas of interest. The curriculum should be structured to fit the needs of medicine rather than to please the students as many curricula have been in the past. And, finally, the faculty and the students should be placed after the care of patients in terms of the system direction.

The control of the number of doctors is essential. Karen Davis (1982) reports that increased numbers of medical school graduates lead directly to increased fees for specialty services, higher physician costs per capita, increased bed demand, increased patient stays, and increased daily costs of hospitals. Tierney (1980) has made some interesting suggestions to restrict physician supply. He recommends a Certificate of Need (CON) for physicians much as we have for hospitals and for large scale equipment. This might take the form of limitation of the number of graduates from medical schools, the control of residencies, limitation of the number of beds in hospitals, increased use of HMOs, direct employment of physicians by the government or the hospital and the operation of incentives to lower physician numbers.

Several writers have stated that there is no correlation between health resources and health manpower and the health status of the country. In fact, there is evidence to suggest that an increment of perhaps 100 percent in funds is necessary to effect a 1 percent improvement in health care. There is no question but that mortality rates have remained essentially constant for 2 or 3 decades despite a doubling and tripling of the health care expenses (Fig. 2).

Attinger (1975) has pointed out that primitive societies believed in a broad definition of health when the shaman served as advisor, physician, teacher, and priest. Modern medicine has become more and more disease-oriented and the highly skilled modern physician has lost a multidimensional concept of health. It is this concept which we must regain. Society invests in a human

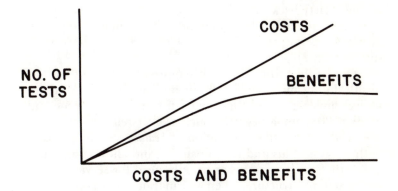

Figure 2.   The relationship between the costs of additional tests performed on a patient and the benefit the patient is likely to receive.

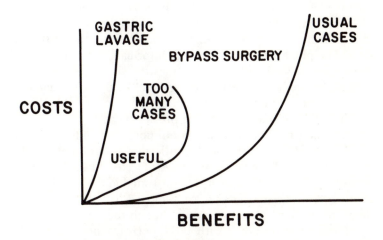

Figure 3.   An extension of Figure 2. A demonstration that the degree of benefit varies widely with the cost of technology and may be negative in some instances.

from birth until age twenty, after which the individual is expected to pay society back until age seventy, after which society must again assume the burden. If an individual is unable to produce during the period of earning because of medical disability, society suffers (Fig. 3).

One of the difficulties of this approach is that indicators of health do not measure health but measure disease. Moreover, we lack any measure of consumer satisfaction and our measures of health rely upon negatives such as over-reliance on surgery. We need an objective description of *health care* that will satisfy both professionals and the consumer and allow comparisons across the system in terms of benefit, need for service, and the socioeconomic structure. Then we can train physicians to render proper care.

## CONTINUING EDUCATION

The newer techniques in medicine arrive daily. New drugs are invented and introduced. The physician must find some way to keep up with this deluge of information and sort from it those ideas which are directly useful. Continuing Education is the answer. The physician is provided with information through formal short courses, through telecommunication via videotapes or television, by medical society meetings, etc. In many specialties a formal amount of education is required, but many of the hours which fulfill the requirement are pro forma at best.

The best method to assure continuous update for the physician is probably a difficult recertification program at regular intervals. Most of the specialties have objected to such a formal approach. The need is clearly demonstrated in the fact that only about 100 physicians per year are removed from the practice of medicine for poor performance, although there must be many more than that number with poor performance among the 450,000 physicians in the country. Very few state medical societies require continuing education for relicensure and only six of the many academies of medicine require recertification (JAMA, 1981) of their members at regular intervals.

## The Consumer

The consumer must be educated in order to develop a system of medical care which provides the best response for the smallest cost. The present consumer tends to assume that tertiary care is the only acceptable method and, in fact, requests hospital care and additional tests beyond those appropriate to the disease. Yet the patient tends to hear and believe ads on television, fails to take prescribed medicines, and does not follow simple instructions. We greatly need a program of education for the consumer, pointing out the system operation, the costs of care, the use of primary systems, and other pertinent details which will reduce the cost of care.

Over and above this type of problem exists a problem in information and communication. The patient usually has little concept of medical procedures and the physician is usually unwilling to take the time to explain fully. As a result, the patient goes into a procedure without a thorough understanding of the risks involved. Several cases brought to the attention of Congress resulted in passage of "informed consent" legislation in which the patient signs a form certifying that he or she has been told of the risks and is aware of the difficulties of the treatment. Despite heroic efforts on the part of the institutional review boards and the federal government, patients remain largely uninformed about what is likely to happen to them in the hospital. Should patients be informed that they are likely to have an iatrogenic disease about 10 percent of the time? Should they be told of the risks of experimental or diagnostic procedures which are often not spelled out?

The patient is becoming aware of this ethical question. As a result there are tens of thousands of malpractice suits in this country every year and the cost of malpractice insurance may be in the thousands of dollars for a surgeon. Admittedly, many of these suits may have little foundation in fact, but the responsibility devolves upon the manager of the system, who may be required to support the physician. The solution may be a better informed public.

The young physician must be licensed to practice medicine.

The license confers a monopoly on the profession and restricts the entrance of outsiders. It permits restriction of practice of the nonlicensed individual and regulates the number of individuals admitted to practice. When the number of physicians increases above comfortable limits, as it does in some states, the restrictions can be made more rigid for licensure and thus permit fewer individuals to practice.

The usual statement made by the profession is that licensure is designed to protect the patient against poor methodology and malpractice. If such were actually the case one would expect to see physicians removed from practice for poor procedures, relicensure of physicians at regular intervals, and a regulation on distribution of physicians in both type and location. The AMA has opposed all of these regulatory measures and the only conclusion which can be reached is that licensure is a form of monopoly and not directly related to the quality of care.

The situation comes to a head in the FMG (Foreign Medical Graduate). Tight restrictions including rigid examinations are required of all physicians who wish to practice in the United States after training in a foreign institution. Physician groups have made it clear that the purpose of the examination is not so much to establish the quality of the physician (although this is of course a criterion) as it is to limit the number of physicians in hospital practice who might infringe upon the monopoly.

*Chapter 3*

# THE PHYSICIAN

The costs of a medical education are miniscule compared to the costs to society after the physician graduates. Current estimations are that the average physician will cost society about $300,000 per year during the rest of that doctor's life. This includes charges to patients out of which must come office expenses, assistants, and personal income. The average physician in private practice nets about $75,000 per year (Owens, 1983). Furthermore, the doctor may increase this income by specialization which adds about 35 percent to the total (Owens, 1983). The physician may decide to become a surgeon, which multiplies the base income two to three times. And it is clear that this additional training does not enhance performance as a practitioner in that up to 40 percent of the practice is usually general practice which could be performed by a much less well trained individual (Spiegel, 1983). Last year physicians had about 600 million office visits for which they received about $11.4 billion under Medicare, while surgeons had only 15 million operations for which they received $4.6 billion.

The average physician has little information on the costs of care. The general assumption is that the physician will provide everything which in this doctor's opinion is best for the patient, and the question of payment may not arise. Third-party payment and the payment of bills retroactively both tend to isolate the physician from the actual costs of services, especially those services rendered in the hospital where most of the costs are incurred.

The retrospective payment method also encourages the protectionism surrounding the average physician. The insurance company will pay for most tests ordered. In the case of Medicare only about 20 percent of bills are refused payment on the basis of overcharges. The physician can order more tests for personal protection rather than for the good of the patient and know that most bills will be honored.

In this regard, it should be pointed out that the physician usually represents about 20–25 percent of the total health care costs in the country and also represents about 80 percent of hospital costs or another 35 percent of the total bill. This occurs because the physician determines who will enter the hospital, the type of care to be provided, the number and type of tests given, and the time which will be spent in the institution. It has been estimated that the hospital contributes about 20 percent of the total amount usually charged to the hospital for services, cleaning, administration, etc.

## How the Physician Uses the System

Many practices of the physician have been under scrutiny. Only a few will be dealt with here and some will recur in other contexts. As we have mentioned, there is a strong possibility that the physician overuses drug prescription orders. In about 75 percent of all ambulatory care visits at least one prescription is provided (Cypress, 1982). In addition, of the drugs prescribed, 75 percent were brand names despite the clear demonstration that generic drugs save money for the patients and are equally effective. Most of the prescriptions were for antihistamines, antibiotics, central nervous system depressants or stimulants, or drugs to control water or calorie intake or loss. Some questions have been raised about how many of these drugs were necessary and how many were to alleviate America's hypochondria. When we realize that 580 million outpatient visits were made last year, there is good reason for the nation's drug bill of $25 billion.

Physicians have been indicted by many economists because of a direct conflict of interest. Many physicians own hospitals, laboratories, drug stores, apparatus manufacturing companies, and the like. Ethicists have proposed that no physicians should own such businesses because the more drugs, lab use, or apparatus required, the more profit the physician makes (Barry, 1982). It is not difficult to reconcile the dilemma of a highly moral physician treating a patient who could resist one more test which might clinch a diagnosis and at the same time double the profit of a visit.

There have been questions about the kind of care given in the United States. When the Teamsters Union had records of its members reviewed by a group of noted authorities, they found that only 27 percent of the care could be counted as good and that much of care rendered was less than adequate (Brook, 1970). A study by the New York Academy of Medicine (1933) suggested that 80 percent of the deaths recorded could be traced to poor medical judgment. These are admittedly older studies and the situation may have improved but they indicate the trends. Studies within the last 3 years have indicated that about 6 percent of physicians at the minimum are drug addicts, alcoholics, or should not be practicing medicine for other reasons (*Family Health*, 1977). In spite of this poor record, the health care bill of the country is increased by about $7 billion per year solely as the cost of defensive medicine which is unnecessary to the treatment of the patient (Tancredi, 1978).

Studies on the use of technology indicate that physicians, in their concern for patient care, often use, at the patient's expense, technology which is worthless. The use of thermography to detect cancer is only about 50 percent effective and has a high number of false positive results (Libshitz, 1978) yet was used extensively for years. Inhalation therapy may actually do more harm than good to many patients but is a part of the hospital armamentarium ordered by many doctors (Gibson, 1974). Carels (1980) has stated that 25 percent of all procedures performed in the care of a patient are unnecessary. The use of radical rather than partial mastectomy, the use of radiotherapy in the treatment of cancer of many types, and the use of clinical laboratory services are other indications of overuse of technology without benefit and perhaps with harm to the patient (Carel, loc. cit.) (Connelly, 1982).

A major problem in treatment lies in a simple economic fact. About 95 percent of the best care can be achieved with little cost and with high efficiency. The remaining 5 percent to confirm a diagnosis or to practice defensive medicine may be very costly and the benefit at the margin is very small. The curve of benefit vs. costs is asymptotic (Fig. 2, see page 39) and unlimited amounts can be spent with little improvement in outcomes.

There are other considerations. The average newborn care unit has a 40 percent occupancy and does not meet expenses. When newborn ICUs are added to this expense, the cost may be very large. The question arises as to whether maternity cases should be lumped into a single unit. In another vein, in one large city, 20 of 97 hospitals did 94 percent of all radiotherapy but all hospitals maintained the capacity. In most hospitals the average number of deliveries per year is about 1,000 and the number required to break even on ob/gyn units is about 1,600 deliveries per year. Obviously charges must be raised in the hospitals to meet the deficits. The statistical distribution of special units is of importance. In Chicago, 3,000 maternity beds is sufficient and if distributed in 45 hospitals would provide adequate local service to the city. However, some 125 hospitals have such services. If we are willing to go one step further and assume that we will take a 1/1,000 chance that a delivery cannot be accommodated, we can lower the number of beds appreciably (Feldstein, 1979). It has been estimated that providing super care for the 1,000th patient in another location would cost much less than providing the unused service. Again, the physician is at fault. The plethora of beds is due largely to the desire of a physician to practice in a given location and to have all services in that location.

The problem of overordering tests is not confined to the laboratory. Patrick (1983) found that only 7 percent of the lumbar spine x-rays taken in emergency rooms were positive and that in most of those the physical examination revealed tenderness, contusions, or other abnormal physical findings which made the diagnosis. Barium enemas are routine orders in many cases of cancer of the cervix or endometrium but to date there has been a zero correlation between x-ray results and extension of the cancer. Of all abdominal x-rays following injury 98 percent are negative (McCook, 1982) and revised protocols for x-rays of patients with extremity injury would save $140 million per year in the country, with a less than 0.5 percent chance of missing a fracture (Brand, 1982). These incidences, which could be multiplied many times, suggest the overuse of facilities for no gain to the patient and little protection for the physician. Other data point up further problems. In one study (Moss, 1981), 27 out of 55 patients were given antibiotics when there were no indications for the drug. Among patients who have lab tests before entering the hospital, 71 percent have those tests repeated in the hospital. While there may be good reason to repeat suspect tests, it is doubtful that this frequency of repetition is necessary (Stump, 1983). Waghon (1983) found that it cost $540,000 in CAT scans to find each case of cerebral aneurysm. Such examples could be repeated endlessly. These few demonstrate the lack of discretion in choosing the kind and number of tests ordered by the physician.

One of the newer technologies is the PET (Positron Emission Tomography) scanner which requires the expenditure of $3–4 million in a cyclotron or other generator of high energy particles. The estimated cost to operate the system is about $1,000 per hour. The usual charges may be about $2,500 per hour but some administrators estimate that $8,000 would be a more realistic figure. The scanner is postulated to be able to detect Alzheimer's disease, a degeneration of the brain cells, for which there is no cure. Is this a reasonable investment in technology?

We must remember that in spite of the advances in technology the dreams of long life may not be realized. Given the rate of cell degeneration especially in the irreplaceable nervous system, it is doubtful that we can hope to have a life span of more than 100 years (George Crile, 1983).

From another viewpoint, it can be argued that physicians take the easy way for themselves and not for the patients. Some 80 percent of deaths occur in the hospital (Maloney, 1983) at the present time. It can be argued that many of these individuals would die happier and easier in the home or in a hospice (Cohen, 1979).

The physician, to many, as revealed by numerous polls, is more of a technician than a psychologist. The doctor spends very few minutes with patients, uses technology in the form of lab results rather than ears, eye, and hands to make diagnosis, and is unaware of the costs of care or of the alternatives to care. More than 80 percent of physicians are unaware of community resources for home care (Carels, 1980) and rely upon the hospital as the almost sole source of patient support. Connelly (1982) states that the physician now uses more than twice as many tests as 7 years ago for the same diseases and virtually the same treatment. This raises again the question of reliance upon testing to solve problems.

## SOME SOLUTIONS

Many solutions have been proposed for the problems mentioned above. Some have been implemented by the Federal Government in the Medicare program and others will be implemented by insurance companies and others as the cost of care increases. The remedies (?) can be lumped into several categories. Many attempt to control costs through:

Control of the system through prospective reimbursement

Control of the hospital through utilization review and payment methods

Control of the physician through PSRO and direct methods

Control of the patient through individual payment plans

Control of all factors through National Health Insurance

We will discuss control of the physicians here and other controls later in the book.

## THE PHYSICIAN'S FEES

The government has for several years attempted to control the charges of the physician by paying for "just and reasonable" charges. There have been major problems. The cost of an operation of the same difficulty may be four times as "just and reasonable" for one physician as for others (Pettigrew, 1981). It has been suggested that rates charged by physicians should be published so that the general public would be aware of the wide variations.

Patients should have confidence that when they enter the doctor's office the charges will be appropriate to the treatment. Nationwide ranges of fees should be established and insurance companies and the government should pay no more than the average for any procedure. By the same token, such rates would be of great advantage to the rural physicians who traditionally make much less than the urban practitioner and this might attract more doctors to rural areas.

Competition should be encouraged. Ginzberg (1982) says that competition in which rates are published and patients have the right to choose the physicians of their choice might broaden choices of Medicare patients and restructure the whole system toward lower rates. Competition does not exist in the health care industry at the present time. The expanding supply of physicians does not lower costs. It leads to more specialization and higher costs and results in competition for hospital space, which results in more building of unnecessary beds. It may also reduce the use of ancillary cheaper personnel and adversely affect the quality of care offered (Ginzburg, 1981). Einsberg (1978) made a most interesting suggestion for controlling the costs of care. He suggested that the physician be billed personally for all unnecessary tests or procedures ordered on a patient. It is also possible that a reduction in the training of lawyers might also reduce medical care because the enormous cost of defensive medicine could be avoided and the savings passed on to the patient.

## MEDICAID MILLS

There has been considerable complaint about so-called Medicaid mills (Mitchell, 1980, 1982). It is true that 60 percent of Medicaid patients are treated by 14 percent of the physicians. However, there is little documentation to suggest poorer care as such; but it is clear that Medicaid physicians spend 20 percent less time with their patients than do general practitioners.

Many of the Medicaid physicians do have very lucrative practices. There are reports of incomes of over $400,000 per year.

Recent pressures on payment whereby the government limits the amount recoverable by the physicians has restricted access to services. In Medicare the government may insist that physicians accept all Medicare patients who come to them or accept none in an attempt to avoid selection of patient on the basis of degree of illness or ability to pay co-payments. The outcry has been great and the plan may not be implemented because of physician pressure.

The Medicaid mills do have certain characteristics which distinguish them from other practices. Cromwell (1981) found several deviations in a large practice handling Medicaid patients. In such practices the physicians were often more poorly trained and fewer were board certified and more were FMGs than in normal practices. But the practice groups made on the average about 30 percent larger incomes than other practitioners in the same area. Because the payment was essentially guaranteed by the government, the charges were higher; $13 vs. $11 per visit, although expenses were the same (about $6 per visit). Furthermore, the Medicaid clinics charged the government allowed UCR (usual, reasonable, and customary) fees which could be higher for the area than for the neighborhood in which they practiced. In addition, the internists who practiced largely on Medicaid patients adopted techniques not in agreement with colleagues in other forms of practice. They gave 42 percent of the patients injections of one form or another, while the normal average was about 16 percent and they spent much less time with patients. They saw more patients in less total time than that expended by other practitioners.

## WHO SHALL LIVE AND WHO SHALL DIE—THE SURGEON

Surgery in the United States is in a crisis. We are graduating perhaps 10 times as many surgeons as necessary from our medical schools. Each of them goes largely into private practice with attendant costs to society. The increase in the number of surgeons, which far outnumbers the growth in population, means that there are more surgeons each year per unit of population. This results in two major problems. In the first place, in order to make a reasonable income, the surgeon must increase fees to make the same income with fewer operations. This results in the better surgeons of the country making two to three times the income of the average general practitioner. The law of economics—supply and demand—does not work in medicine. As additional surgeons are trained, applications of the law should result in decreased prices for surgery. As noted above, this does not occur and shows no signs of occurring. Secondly, as the number of operations performed by a given surgeon decreases, his or her skill also decreases and mortality increases (Bunker, 1978). Finally, in order to maintain income, the surgeon is forced to do more surgery than is warranted by the medical circumstance. All of these factors are to the detriment of the system.

Numerous examples can be cited. The surgeon often becomes convinced of the advantage of a surgical procedure and begins to use it before it has been medically evaluated. The cardiac bypass operation is a typical example. We now perform about 200,000 bypass operations per year in the United States at a cost of about $15,000 each, not counting morbidity, loss of time from work, etc. The evidence is by no means clear that the procedure is effective. Perhaps 40 percent are clearly benefited. The rest may have some relief from pain but are still incapacitated to some degree. The evidence is also clear that many of these individuals can be treated by drugs alone without operations and do equally well (Bunker, 1978; Wennberg, 1978; Bendixen, 1978) (Fig. 3, see page 39).

One may argue that the operations were necessary in the judgment of the physician and this, in fact, is the argument often used. However, it is difficult to explain the fact that about one-third of all tissues removed at surgery are found to be normal by the pathologist (Sparling, 1962). It is hard to justify operations when the variability is so great. In the state of Vermont alone, where the population and the climate are relatively uniform, the number of hysterectomies ranges from 21 to 60 per 10,000 patients, the mastectomies range from 16 to 35 per 10,000 and the prostatectomies range from 15 to 30 for the same population unit in the various areas of the state (Bendixen, 1978). Some of the surgery performed actually decreases the life span rather than augments it. Surgical survivors of cholecystectomies (removal of the gall bladder) actually survive for a shorter period of time than those patients treated by drugs alone and there is some suggestion that twice as many individuals develop cancer of the large bowel. Hysterectomy in the absence of cancer increases the life span of an individual about 2 weeks (Dyck, 1977). Patients without cancer who have a prostatectomy live about 9 years less than those patients who do not have the operation (Wennberg, 1978).

Of greater concern, surgeons in our day of complicated operations experiment in their surgical procedures about 40 percent of the time and a sizable percentage of the experiments are to the detriment of the patient. Simply put, the surgeon attempts to make revision in the methods of surgery developed by previous experience and this may not be an improvement.

The relationship between the economy and the surgeon is clearcut in other cases. Roos (1983) has mentioned that when a new surgeon moves into a neighborhood the number of surgical operations performed increases about 17 percent even though there are no documented increases in need or incidence of disease.

It is for these reasons that proposals have been made by George Crile of the Cleveland Clinic (1982) that no surgeon be allowed to practice as an individual. Dr. Crile has proposed that to avoid conflict of interest every surgeon should be salaried and employed by a hospital. However, this is not entirely satisfactory. Such a move would restrict the desire to increase income by more surgery; but at the same time the hospital has pressures to maintain usage of operating suites and fill beds and might put pressure on the physician to do more surgery.

Another dilemma faces the medical system with respect to surgery. As new techniques of anesthesia and life maintenance are developed, the surgical procedures become more and more complicated. We are now transplanting kidney, livers, hearts, pancreases, as well as hips and other joints. As each procedure is developed and practiced by more and more surgeons two major problems arise. In the first place, there is a question of quality. Unless the open heart surgical team performs at least two major operations a week (and only about 30 percent of open heart units do so), the risk of mortality is three times that of units performing more operations (Bunker, 1981). One can argue that the team must learn and develop in order to attract more cases and therefore become proficient, but is it worth the life of patients when the need is not clearly demonstrated? Secondly, the cost is rapidly becoming prohibitive. The total cost of a liver transplant is estimated to be about $200,000 before the surgery and many hundreds of thousands after the event. A heart transplant costs about $100,000, a kidney $35,000, and this does not take into account the fact that many patients never return to a useful life, many are sustained at high costs on drugs, and many are a burden to society during a relatively short postoperative life (Table II).

Several means can be adopted to change the surgical situation in the country. First and foremost, we need to restrict the number of medical students who are allowed to practice surgery. Surgery classes might be decreased in the curriculum of medical school, fewer residencies could be offered, and tougher exams could be given. In the ultimate situation it might be possible to refuse payment to surgeons unless the treatment has been approved by a general practitioner or an internist before the operation. Secondly, we could require a second opinion on all surgery before any insurance or Medicare claims were made. It has been clearly demonstrated that second opinions will reduce surgery at least 15 percent (House Committee on Interstate and

**Table 2   Some Examples of the Costs of High Technology in Medicine**

| Technology | Number | Original Costs For Procedures | Continuing Costs Year* | Number Benefited |
|---|---|---|---|---|
| Kidney Transplants | 23,000 | $35,000 | $1,000 | 31% survive 5 yrs. |
| Heart | 500 | $100,000 | $10,000 year | 42% survive 5 yrs. |
| Liver | 540 | $200,000 | $15,000 year | 39% survive 1 yr. |
| Heart | 334 | $50,000 | $5,000 | 25% function well |
| Lung | 38 | $150,000 | $10,000 | 10 months survival |
| Heart Lung | 22 | $90,000 | $10,000 | ? |
| Bone Marrow | 2,000 | $100,000 | $10,000 | 50% cure est. |
| Bypass, Cardiac | 200,000 | $20,000 | $2,000 | 60% Improved |
| Pacemaker | 400,000(?) | $5,000 | 5-yr. or sooner replacement | 25% have defects |
| Renal Dialysis | 50,000(?) | ———— | $25,000 year | 5-yr. survival |

*Continuing costs represent costs of immunosuppression with cyclosporin or other drugs, repeated dialysis or similar costs, and maintenance in terms of maintaining correct electrolyte balances, etc.
Original costs include surgery, crossmatching of tissues, preparations, tests, etc.

Foreign Commerce, 1976). Surgeons object to a second opinion on the basis of cost, or the fact that the second opinion may not be any better than the first and reflects on their judgment. The evidence points out that second opinion does work and does reduce surgeries.

Another proposal suggests that surgeons be concentrated in hospitals which would specialize in only one service (say kidney transplants) so that the best talent could be gathered together in one place and the lowest cost offered to the patient (Carels, 1980). In one respect this is already being achieved. "Same-day surgery" is springing up over the country. For those relatively minor operations which require anesthesia but not complicated apparatus such as heart-lung bypass equipment (hernia, tonsil, etc.) the patient enters in the morning, has surgery and is discharged in the afternoon. The procedure is cheap, safe, and effective. Surgeons in private practice object strongly to the method, on the basis that accidents or untoward events may occur which would require sophisticated apparatus. Questions are also raised about the competence of surgeons operating such a "fly-by-night" situation. The evidence is against the medical societies and the surgeons. The outpatient surgery has proven to be effective and safe. Similar questions have been raised on the establishment of outpatient emergency clinics which are operated by surgeons under salary to a large corporation and which charge much less than hospital emergency departments. Again the objections are that such isolated stations do not have the backup of a large hospital. Again the evidence is against the hospital and the surgeons in that the stand-alone clinics are providing safe and effective service.

The Health Care Financing Administration has also proposed that the fees for hospital-based physicians be 60 percent of that of office-based doctors in order to correct for the cost of maintaining an office. The proposal has also been made that Medicare patients be required to go to the cheapest doctor and doctors be allowed to bid for patients. As HCFA states the case, there is no reason for a difference of from $8,200 to $2,100 charged for the same procedure on the same type of patient.

Some 30 percent of American physicians consider themselves to some degree specialists in surgery, and about a fourth of those beginning residency training are going into surgical programs. At the Harvard Medical School, Osler L. Peterson and his colleagues undertook to find out just who are doing surgery in the U.S. and how much they do, and whether fewer surgeons could handle the load. Their conclusions have been published in *The New England Journal of Medicine:* Too many physicians of all kinds are performing operations, and most of them—even many of the best-trained ones, thoroughly committed to surgery—have modest workloads.

Peterson examined hospital records in four metropolitan regions and noted the operations performed by each physician.

Each operation was weighted on an index that had been devised by the California Medical Association according to its complexity and the time required for preoperative and postoperative care: For example, a normal delivery or a tonsillectomy had a weight of 4, an appendectomy a weight of 9.5, and the repair of an abdominal aortic aneurysm a weight of 40. The total weighted workload of each of 2,700 physicians was aggregated for the year. The largest workloads recorded for surgical specialists who had been certified by their specialty board had a medial "California relative value" equivalent to about 180 "typical" operations a year. The operating load of self-described surgical specialists lacking board certification was only 60 percent as great; that of general practitioners with a secondary specialty in surgery was less than 20 percent of the board-certified surgeons' load. Other general practitioners, osteopathic physicians, and medical specialists (internists, pediatricians, cardiologists, and so on) did far fewer operations a year.

A large fraction of the physicians did very few operations a year and a small fraction did many. There was a wide variation in workloads. Thirty-one percent of the 2,700 physicians who did operations had California-relative-value loads of 50 (equivalent to five appendectomies) or less; 14 percent had loads of 2,000 (equivalent to 210 appendectomies or more). As might be expected, the less specialized physicians do fewer and less complex operations, but the variation in load was large even among board-certified surgical specialists. The busiest 10 percent of them did more than 350 typical operations a year and the least busy 25 percent of them did fewer than about 100 a year. A special analysis revealed that it takes a long time to build up a surgical practice to even a modest workload. A study of 780 surgical specialists who had graduated from medical school no more than 25 years before showed that it had taken them about 18 years to reach their maximum operating load and about 13 years to reach 90 percent of that maximum.

What if the operating load were redistributed? If only surgical specialists did all operations except the very simplest ones, their workload would be increased by 16 percent, or by about two operations a month. If the operations done by specialists who in 1970 had loads of fewer than 50 operations a year were distributed among those who did more work, the mean load of those busier specialists would increase 20 percent. If surgical operations were limited to board-certified surgeons, the operating load of those surgeons would be increased by 57 percent to just over 300 operations a year, or about six a week.

These data suggest that not only do we have too many surgeons but that many of them are performing at a level where it is impossible to maintain skills. The solutions are obvious. Fewer medical students should be trained in surgery, only board certified surgeons should be allowed to practice, second opinions should be required for every procedure except very minor ones and some system of fee schedules should be established to inform the patient of the probable costs.

## SUMMARY

As we look across the medical field several general principles come to light. On the whole, physicians believe that the use of more resources will improve service, whereas the contrary may actually be true. Physicians use resources in order to protect themselves, to satisfy patient demand for service, and to make more money. The demand for service and the surplus of physicians and surgeons, together with the payment by retrospectives charges and through third-party payers has increased costs of care. These factors suggest that some changes are possible. The most logical steps to rearrange the system would be to publish the fees and costs of care, to use the prospective payment system, to refuse to pay for unnecessary tests, to place an absolute ceiling on costs by paying all physicians the same for equal work and to provide an educational service for the physicians. One suggestion is that the physicians be provided with a copy of the patient's bill with all charges clearly stated. Another step in the right direction would be a refusal to pay for a specialist unless needed and requested by a general practitioner.

These maneuvers are not likely to be accepted by the medical profession within the foreseeable future. And that is too bad, for in these measures lies one method of controlling health care costs.

Burnham, writing in *Science* (1982), pointed out that medicine went through a golden age in the 1960s when the image was Dr. Kildare and Marcus Welby. Physicians were heroes in the movies and on the battlefield. In the 1970s and to the present, that picture has changed. The physician is pictured as charging excessive fees, indulging in unethical acts, performing unnecessary procedures, and running a business rather than a profession. Lists of criticisms include failure to take a personal interest in the patient, unavailability in an emergency, long waiting times in offices, and failure to communicate. In addition to these social criticisms, we are now beginning to hear greater complaints about incompetence in the actual practice of medicine. The physician must be aware of the attitudes and work to change them.

*Chapter 4*

# CONTROL OF THE SYSTEM

Because of the billions of dollars of taxpayers' money invested yearly in Medicaid and Medicare, the Federal Government has been greatly concerned about the control of costs of health care. Because of the difficulty of controlling the fees and operations of 300,000 physicians, attempts first were made to control the 6,000 hospitals. The original control systems on physicians were on the group as a whole through PSRO (Professional Services Review Organizations). At a later date it became obvious that a major culprit in rising costs was the retrospective payment system. HMO (Health Maintenance Organization) and PPO (Preferred Provider Organizations) were encouraged to control costs and a prospective payment system was adopted for hospitals. That system will soon be extended to the physician.

Each of the systems has advantages and disadvantages. In general, the advantages outweigh the disadvantages. Most of the systems have been put into place over the objections of the American Medical Association and the county Medical Societies.

## The HMO

An HMO is an organization that accepts contractual responsibility for making available and providing to all enrollees a specified range of medical care services at an identified location in return for their prepaid capitation payments. A cardinal feature of the HMO premium is that it is paid by each enrollee before services are used and regardless of the volume or type of covered services actually provided. The HMO operation budget derives entirely from prepaid capitation payments, supplemented by additional premiums and cost-sharing fees. The organization thus assumes prospective financial risk for producing all services demanded by enrollees during the contract period and usually for reimbursement of payments made by the enrollee for services provided outside the HMO area in emergency situations (Lewis, 1976).

Two forms of the HMO model have been recognized. The centralized form of HMO is usually called the prepaid group practice. In a typical arrangement the subscriber pays monthly premiums for comprehensive health care services which are provided by an organized medical group. The largest and probably best known HMO is the Kaiser-Permanente program which serves 2.2 million members in California, Oregon, Colorado, and Ohio (Saward, 1973).

The decentralized form of an HMO is encompassed by the term Foundation for Medical Care (FMC). The best known HMO of this type is the San Joaquin Foundation for Medical Care, founded by that county's medical society. This foundation combines a pre-payment mechanism for patients with fee-for-service solo practice for the physicians. The FMC is an agency that enrolls physicians who agree to a central billing mechanism, peer review of quality, and cost control. It then contracts, usually with employers and/or unions health and welfare funds, to provide a stipulated package of health care benefits to covered persons in return for a per-person payment to the FMC from the contracting entity. The physician bills the FMC for services rendered.

When HMOs were first proposed, they were hailed as the answer to the lack of preventive medicine and the cost containment by the existing medical health care system. Broad coverage of ambulatory care, as well as hospitalization, was believed to encourage preventive services and early detection of illness, since patients could seek care early in an episode with few financial or supply restraints, and physicians could act to avert later and far more costly hospitalization.

In the prepaid system the physician is compensated by a payment fixed in advance and is usually required to absorb additional costs and may retain additional fees if costs are lower than expected. The physician in the HMO thus has a marked incentive to provide less tertiary care with expensive add-ons and to encourage preventive medicine to avoid undue expenses. Fee-for-service physicians, on the other hand, reduce their income if they practice this type of medicine, and, in fact, the system encourages them to provide additional services, to encourage multiple visits, and to disregard costs in determining procedures to be followed.

The truth lies somewhere in between. The quality of care provided in the HMO is equivalent to fee-for-service care. There is little evidence of skimping on care. After all, patients dissatisfied with care can withdraw at will, so it is in the HMO's best interests to provide excellent care. The charge of recruiting selected populations is probably true. HMOs have enrolled members of unions, factory work forces, etc., who are healthier than the general public.

The HMO has been challenged in many states, particularly in Texas, as an example of the corporate practice of medicine. Medical societies have fought the establishment of HMO across the country as a direct interference in the private practice of medicine. This is a little difficult to understand when we realize that 90 percent of the present graduating classes in medical school indicate that they intend to go into group practice (Cypress, 1983). Although group practice is still legally fee-for-service, which is acceptable to the medical societies, the trend is slowly moving toward HMO type practices. Several million people are now covered by a technique of medical practice known as the PPO (Preferred Provider Organization). In this type of practice the subscriber pays a flat rate per year for service and may go to any doctor or hospital in the plan for service. Since each doctor is paid on the basis of the patients which come to him or her,

her, the doctor sees the practice as a fee-for-service payment. If the patient does not elect to go to a doctor or hospital in the plan, 20 percent will be added to the bill. The largest plan at the moment is the Mountain Medical Affiliate in Colorado which has 160,000 subscribers. The AMA has not yet taken a firm position but is suspected to oppose the idea.

## THE PSRO AS A CONTROL DEVICE

Another attempt to control the system resulted in the creation of a professional standard review organization (PSRO). As the federal outlay for health care rose more than a billion dollars a year from 1969 to 1975 and monthly premium costs of Medicare increased, more and more concern over control developed. The great cost increase was due to two factors—increase in unit cost of service and increase in the number of services. A major objective of any health care system must be containment of utilization of services, and this implies some form of control. Although Medicare required utilization review from the beginning, these reviews were at best cursory. There was little professional participation.

In an attempt to remedy the review process for Medicare, the PSRO legislation (PL-92-603) was enacted on October 30, 1972. The law required designation of PSROs over the entire country. They were required to represent physicians of all types. Participation was voluntary, but if medical groups refused to organize, the secretary of DHEW could designate other groups to form the PSRO.

A PSRO is expected to determine if the services provided are both necessary and up to standard, including review of service, hospital admission, length of stay, and the necessary services. The PSRO role becomes critical when one realizes that present estimates are that the costs of Medicare will overrun older estimates by $240 billion in 20 years. The overrun is due to the increase in the number of services provided to beneficiaries. According to a Senate Finance Committee Report in September 1972, a significant portion of such services proved to be unnecessary. Utilization review was found not to be satisfactory and, in fact, was effective only when hospital beds were in short supply.

The PSRO is charged with responsibility to determine whether care and services were appropriate for the disease in accord with professional standards for all Medicare patients. In order to take advantage of size and the lowered administrative expense for computers and other such equipment associated with larger size, PSROs are organized only where a substantial number of physicians are available, at least 300 in a group. Participation is voluntary and open to all physicians.

One of the first problems to arise was the setting of standards for acceptable medical care. The guidelines for use of antibiotics, screening procedures, and so forth, are being developed by professional associations. It will eventually be necessary to set guidelines for almost all medical and surgical treatment, which may require years. The present standard is "reasonable" care, and varies from physician to physician and state to state.

Problems with PSROs are centered in a gray area where health services research has not yet provided satisfactory answers. Before PSROs can be truly successful, we must develop:

> The measures for efficacy of present medical technique;
>
> The cost-to-benefit ratio of various modes of treatment;
>
> A nationwide system for assessing quality of care to adjust inequalities; and
>
> A method for quality assurance evaluation.

Two kinds of political solutions are likely. As more and more patients come under the same form of insurance funded by the government, more physicians will be forced to accede to review. Second, as more medical organizations, such as the American College of Family Practice, require recertification at regular intervals, review may be a necessity for continuing certification.

The PSRO, when properly applied, does work. The Forward Plan for Health, 1978–82 (DHEW) documents that a 20 percent reduction in hospital stay was achieved by one PSRO. Another found that seeking a second opinion on the need for surgery reduced cases by 29 percent. Many other similar cases could be cited. The intended extension of PSRO to long-term and ambulatory care could produce even greater effects.

The need for PSROs has been based on the need for review of quality of health care. Quality of review may be determined by several factors:

*Need:* (Ertel, 1977) In Kansas, elective surgery rates varied from 74 to 24 per 10,000 in various regions; infection rates in hospitals varied from zero to 24 per 1,000 and justified hysterectomies from 20 to 80 percent from one hospital to another. Similar findings have been reported from Vermont, Alabama, and elsewhere. This suggests the need for setting national standards of care. Yet physicians claim they can monitor and control such discrepancies.

*Costs:* There appears to be no question that costs of PSRO review increase health costs. It costs about $15 per patient stay to obtain a PSRO evaluation, and highly trained personnel are required. A study of savings from shorter stays, better diagnosis, and so forth indicates that the PSRO system may pay its own way (Ertel, 1977) after starting costs are met.

*Interference:* Physicians often claim that PSROs interfere with the practice of medicine "in the way they practice it." Claims are also made that sample size does not permit adequate review. The average physician sees 2,000 patients per year, not enough to evaluate treatment for rare diseases. Second, few providers in an age of specialization are responsible for the patient over a period of time, so total treatment cannot be evaluated.

*Measurements:* There is not yet enough experience to determine the criteria for evaluation in many cases. When the medical audit is well applied, it is very effective. Reports indicate a major increase in effectiveness of appendicitis diagnosis (disease pathology rose from 18 to 55 percent and antibiotic use declined from 60 to 30 percent in the same period.) New approaches to PSRO review deal with diagnostic outcomes and final outcome of treatment.

*Data Base:* In order to have an effective professional standards review organization, it is necessary to accumulate a large data base on which to base projection of quality and care and utilization. The Texas Medical Foundation (TMF) is now operating a large Medicare program for the state of Texas to set such criteria.

*Provider Domination:*     There is a real risk of the "old boy" syndrome developing in PSROs. Only time will answer this question. There is no question but that PSRO has been effective in some locations, but the countrywide experience is negligible.

The PSRO constitutes a control system in which feedback to the physician's action is the comment of the review panel. In those circumstances in which criteria were set by active participation of the physicians involved, feedback works very well. However, experience has shown that only 10 to 20 percent of professionals will participate in setting standards, and the immediate response of any physician to criticism at not setting standards is to question their validity.

When this happens, masses of data are collected, but if the physicians do not use the data to improve performance, the effort is wasted and, in the parlance, the loop is open. In Utah, it became clear that when physicians' compliance with the criteria was 70 percent or less, they questioned criteria rather than their own performance.

Ultimately, the effectiveness of the PSRO is a function of the effectiveness of medical care. The measurement of outcomes then becomes a major problem. A PSRO should be able to determine if the outcome of a treatment was favorable and, if unfavorable, to modify treatment. This is difficult. The individual may not see more than a few patients with a given disease in a lifetime, so statistics mean little. The costs per patient are too high ($15) to follow every patient, so only a random sample can be selected. If specialists are used, as is customary, responsibility is divided and the statistical base is eroded. All of these are problems that must be directly addressed if PSRO is to be successful.

As a part of a political system, the PSRO must fulfill certain criteria that have not been previously necessary with a group of doctors practicing a mild form of self-policing. These conditions are:

> A hard data base must be accumulated to back up decisions on practice.
>
> There must be peer consensus on the standards adopted.

Public accountability is necessary.

Internal validity is critical for good standards of care.

An external sponsor for the PSRO must be assured to reduce bias.

As an essentially political arm of both the government and the county medical society, the PSRO* must fill several roles: it must be the accountable agent for health quality; it must maintain an educational base to change attitudes; it must evaluate progress; it must be a means of communication; and, it is hoped it will serve both as an innovator and as a legal protection device against malpractice.

It should be clear that several different functions have been implied above. **Utilization review** is a concurrent process that looks at the cost of medical care and makes adjustments by allocating medical service (kinds of service, need for service) and by determining the appropriateness of service. The **medical audit** looks mainly at quality of service and assesses the performance of a provider as a control on quality. It is retrospective in nature. **Medical care evaluation** looks at patterns of disease to determine methodology of treatment; it is concerned mostly with analysis of aggregate sources of data and errors of the system.

In summary, a major problem in the health care system is the assessment of the quality of care and correction of any deficits which may be discovered. Problems are rooted in the mores of the medical profession which resents the possible intrusion of outside reviewers into the process of medical care delivery.

### REIMBURSEMENT

Prospective reimbursement is a method of paying hospitals amounts or rates of payment that are determined in advance for the coming year. These amounts or rates, regardless of the cost actually incurred, are paid to the hospital. This method of reimbursement is attracting the interest of policy makers and purchasers, both public and private, as a method of combating rise in hospital cost.

---

* Newer parlance uses PSO rather than PSRO

About 35 prospective reimbursement systems were currently in operation across the nation in 1976. Blue Cross Plans operated 22, nine are operated by state agencies or commissions and several by state hospital associations (Dowling, 1976). Participation by hospitals in Blue Cross and hospital association programs is generally voluntary, whereas participation in state programs is mandatory. Blue Cross prospective reimbursement systems affect only what hospitals are paid for their patients, while state systems differ with regard to who must pay the rates set by the agency or commission. In some states, Medicaid reimburses the costs only to patients who pay billed charges with Blue Cross. In other states, Blue Cross and Medicaid pay the approval rates. However, no state has jurisdiction over the federal Medicare program.

The objectives of prospective reimbursement are to establish an agreed upon rate for all payers prior to the rendering of service, allow hospitals to set a budget and charge patients based on this budget before the year begins, and to operate within that budget (Dowling, 1976).

The objectives set by the bodies for prospective reimbursement programs are to establish macroeconomic controls, encourage better management, discourage underutilization, rationalize facility and program expansions, and also to encourage better patient management by discouraging excessive lengths of stay for selected diagnostic categories.

Prospective reimbursement systems can function properly if the fiscal officers in the hospitals can:

*Adopt uniform chart of accounts*    in order to provide the prospective reimbursement system commission with comparable data to review conflicts with responsibility accounting and in consistency in recording data for Medicare.

*Adopt uniform statistical procedures*    in order to provide the commission with comparable data that will define the productivity statistics and cost allocation statistics on a uniform basis.

*Adopt new budget forms*   in order to provide same form for all hospitals to use when submitting budgets to the commission.

*Prepare for budgeting.*   Prior to preparing the next fiscal year's budget it is necessary to include prior year revenues, expenses, productivity statistics on the budget forms, complete the cost allocations and compute the unit cost and unit revenue for each revenue department for each year.

*Monitor Compliance.*    During the budget year, it will be necessary for the fiscal officer to monitor compliance with the commission approved plan.

*Adopt Uniform Annual Reporting.*    After the end of the budget year, it will be necessary to prepare financial reports on uniform forms provided by the commission. This report is generally public information and available to whoever requests it.

The basis of payment used in prospective reimbursement may include:

Total hospital budget
Departmental budgets
Family or person (Capitation)
Care or stay
Day charges
Specific services

The impact of prospective reimbursement on hospital operation depends upon type of basis of payment used by the hospital. The areas of hospital performance that might be affected by prospective reimbursement can be identified by the factors that determine costs in hospitals. The following is proposed as a complete although general list of these cost-influencing factors (Lewis & Howard, 1977):

Cases treated
Case mix
Length of stay
Scope of service
Amenity level
Quality level
Efficiency
Input prices

Investment in the maintenance or improvement of human
   physical resources
Teaching programs

The total hospital budget, departmental budget, or capitation bases of payment encourages reduction in cases treated and length of stay of hospitalized patients, because the amounts to be paid under these payment units are set and they would not be affected by admission or patient days of care provided. A hospital would simply receive each month the third-party payer's share of one-twelfth of the total amount agreed to pay for the year. As a result, hospitals might attempt to admit more selectively and to discharge patients sooner to alternative facilities, or to their homes, or might develop pre-admission testing, out-patient surgery, out-patient diagnostic and treatment services, and home care programs to prevent or shorten hospitalization.

In addition to means of reducing admission and patient days, hospitals might admit fewer complex or serious cases, thereby shifting toward less costly case mix. Also, hospitals could discontinue or delay costly programs and services thereby reducing the scope of service they offer. All of these actions tend to moderate increases in expenditures for equipment, personnel, supplies and hence act in the direction of keeping actual costs below prospective budget.

The case, the days of stay, and the specific services payment units are all output related. In general, the use of any of these output measures as the basis of payment would motivate hospitals to increase the quantity of that output and to contain the quality level, intensity, and scope of service provided per unit of output to increase efficiency, and to contain input prices, investments in resources, and teaching programs, all of which act in the direction of reducing the cost per unit of output. Payment of a fixed amount per day would motivate hospitals to increase the days of care provided by increasing admissions and lengths of stay.

Payment of fixed amounts for specific services such as nursing care, laboratory tests, surgical procedures, and X-rays will motivate hospitals to provide more services. The number of patients requiring services might be increased by increasing admissions and lengths of stay or hospitals might attempt to admit the more complex case type, since they need the most services.

To be acceptable, prospective reimbursement must result in budgets or rates that meet the financial requirements of hospitals. Also, rates should apply equally to patients and third-party payers. Since the factors of utilization, service intensity, and technology are major factors in rising hospital expenditures, one must look beyond the reimbursement rate itself for better ways of decreasing utilization and directly limiting supply.

Since reimbursement by third parties has become a major source of capital funds, hospitals can only be expected to accept prospective reimbursement if they believe that rates will be set high enough to assure the capital funds they believe they need. Consideration of capital needs could also be met if the hospital is operating at efficiency level. For example, hospitals that could contain costs might accrue surpluses gained, by keeping actual costs below prospective rates. Under such an approach, a hospital that is efficient relative to comparable hospitals could use the earned surpluses for new facilities or services.

Development of variable prospective budgets or rates for different use levels, such as separate fixed and variable costs would allow for other kinds of unexpected events, for example, equipment breakdowns, unexpected volume, and union wages settlements which must be accommodated by adjusting the rates.

## The DRG

Fetter (1980) has presented the case for Diagnostic Review Groups (DRG) very well. The payers for medical care have always been in a dilemma. Charges have been based on bed costs and additional charges. Furthermore, costs and charges bear no relationship to each other and some patients are billed by one method and some by another depending upon the payer. It is obvious that every patient does not have the same charges for services and that some diseases require much more intensive care than others. An attempt to adjust the costs leads to the concept of prospective payment, but although this method controls costs to some extent, it is still based on the old standards of care and does not take into consideration the actual costs of service. As a result, the concept of DRG has arisen. The basic idea is simple. Diseases with about the same services and costs are lumped into groups and the average cost of treatment is determined. Rastuccia (1980) found, for example, that for a neoplasm the average cost was $2,700, while the cost was $801 for ear diseases, $3,100 for acute myocardial infarction, and the average for all disease was about $1,400. In grouping patients by disease, the system takes in account 23 major categories such as nervous system, eye, gastrointestinal disease, and other similar categories. Within each category a breakdown is possible depending upon age of the patient, whether an operation is necessary, and the severity of the disease. The diseases are classified by a standard method, the ICD (International Disease Classification) which has as many as 7,000 classifications. The system can be illustrated with a simple case. A patient admitted with ulcer may stay 6 days on medical treatment, 11 days with endoscopy, and 17 days with gastric resection. The first category uses only 13 percent of the resources used by the last. A DRG would take such differences into account.

The American Medical Association developed over a period of time the PAS (Professional Activity Study), which is essentially a study of length of stay for many disease classifications based on the ICD codes. This system has been used by PSROs in evaluation studies of performance of physicians and hospitals.

The concept of DRG began with the PAS study but recognized the complexity of the 7,000 entities to be classified and attempted to simplify the procedures. Their criteria were simple. Any definition

Must be medically clear

Must be defined in variables which can be obtained from the patient records

Must have a manageable number of classes (500 were chosen)

Must have similar outcomes within each class

The major criterion was the LOS (Length of Stay). The LOS was calculated for each category of disease based on retrospective hospital data and all prospective admissions were admitted based on the average LOS. There are obviously difficulties. Some hospitals have a much longer LOS than others for the same disease. However, the data would permit questioning the physician about a stay which was too short or too long compared to others in the same hospital but it would not permit the assignment of an average stay for the whole country. Extension of the DRG to the entire country would greatly serve to equalize the length of stay across the country.

Each category of disease could also be assigned a cost based on LOS and services rendered. Knowing the average costs for a given disease would permit tighter control on the costs of treatment.

The state of New Jersey has been implementing DRG in the form of SHARE (Standard Hospital Accounting and Rate Evaluation) for some time. New Jersey has added another feature to those described above. There are disincentives in the form for nonpayment for the excessive use of high technology and costly tests. Indications are that the system may save the state some 20 percent of its hospital costs.

The system must be expanded in two directions. We must avoid per diem costs or charges for the reasons explained above and we must adopt a system of payment for actual needed services, and the system must be extended to the physician in terms of cost of treatment, number of office visits, etc., for particular disease entities.

As we continue to develop systems of DRGs, a change in the patient record will become essential. In order to relate costs and disease categories, a *problem oriented patient record* (POR) becomes invaluable. The ability to diagnose and enter upon the record the problems of the patient makes it much simpler for the person coding for a DRG to locate the disease, the treatment and the diagnosis and to predict the possible outcomes. The POR as developed by Weed and others has not become as widespread in the medical system as it should mainly because the physician is used to entering records by chronological order rather than by problem. As a result the present medical record is incomplete, inaccurate, and often unreadable. The POR automatically places events in relation to the problems of the patient and relates treatment to each of the problems.

The overall goals of the DRGs are to provide equitable payment to hospitals, encourage efficiency of operations, simplify reporting procedures and help in the provision of care for Medicare patients. The design is relatively simple: The plans will be phased in over a 3-year period with rates determined in advance and not controlled by any previous level of expenditure. The reimbursement will be based on nine census regions and on urban and rural categories of services. Several objections occur: The System does not handle typical cases of over or under expense; it is based on a strictly statistical judgment and thus may present inequities.

A commission has been set up to identify medically appropriate patterns for the use of health resources, to assess treatment by new procedures, and to establish the increase in payments due each year as a result of inflation. In addition, each hospital is required to submit to PRO (Professional Review Organization) reviews of admissions, discharges, and quality of care. The hospitals will be expected to treat only those cases in which they have the most expertise and reduce the number of those in which the expertise is below average, which, in turn, will create more specialty hospitals.

It is apparent that the establishment of such review procedure and tight controls on medical costs will require closer cooperation between the hospital and the staff physicians in the use of resources and in the type of medicine practiced.

## The Structure of the DRG

The structure of the practice of medicine has been divided into 23 major diagnostic categories (MDC) and into medical and surgical areas. The 23 large groups have been divided into 467 subgroups based on diagnosis, secondary diagnosis, age, possible complications, and whether or not surgery is required.

The DRGs are based on the approximately 7,000 ICD (International Code of Diseases) codes, which, in turn, are clearly identified by number and by description and which are accepted internationally.

As an example, there are 13 major DRGs for disorders of the eye. These, in turn, are divided into subareas by procedure and diagnosis, which reflect the areas of the eye where disease occurs and the diagnosis based on type of disease (infection, neurological disorder, etc.) and age of the patient. From this information a length of stay is calculated together with the standard deviation from the mean.

The operation of the DRG system is a twofold manipulation of the data. The clinical information is arranged by an expert and a DRG assignment is made. At the same time charges and similar data are merged with the clinical data and the revenue per DRG is calculated. There are problems with both of these streams of data. Some DRGs occur in so few instances that the calculation of a cost factor is impossible. Secondly, the IOM has estimated that 27 percent of all patient records had major errors in clinical information which may increase the costs. These two factors imply that the hospital payment is subject to data accuracy and a failure to collect information on occurrence and costs. Furthermore, surgery DRGs tend to categorize patients into more complex cases and therefore higher costs. Finally, the DRG concept penalizes the hospital with severe cases in higher proportion than the average as they will be paid only for the average case cost. On the other hand, one major advantage of the DRG system will be improvement in medical records. The in-depth review of medical records required for assignment will require better record keeping and higher accuracy and the typing of the fiscal or the clinical data will require timely updating of records and close control of reporting channels.

To date, the major source of errors in DRG assignments can be listed as:

>    Incomplete data
>    Poor documentation of records
>    Failure to use ICD lists
>    Incorrect reporting (coding, sequencing, coding, etc.)
>    Acceptance of telephone calls for clinical information

The hope of the DRG proponents is that the system will result in better patient management both for the hospital and the physician. Admitting practices will be subject to scrutiny, lengths of stay will be monitored, and the physician will be required to keep better records. For the hospital, the DRG will require a better service product analysis, will require strategies for patient admission, and will change physician recruiting practices. Both will be required to look more closely at performance and more efficient scheduling of tests and a more efficient allocation of duties among paraprofessionals and professionals. Hospitals will be forced into joint plans for purchasing and inventory management.

Although we have discussed the DRG with respect to the hospital and the physician, it must be emphasized that it also applies to the other members of the health care team. Nurses will be affected to a considerable extent. Hospitals are likely to resort to variable staffing in order to minimize the number of nurses needed at any given moment. Nurses will be required to monitor more carefully patient stay, medications, and services. The team approach to medical care will be more fully implemented and the nurses will become stronger members of the team. It will be necessary to establish workloads for nurses in accordance with the particular DRG and to estimate time required for the treatment of various DRGs. As hospitals orient

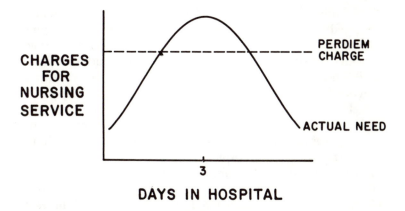

Figure 4.    The cost benefit of paying nurses by the actual need for patient care rather than by the usual per diem rate.

their activities to adopt particular DRGs and decrease emphasis on others, the number or type of use of nurses may change radically in individual units (Fig. 4).

The TEFRA (Tax Equity and Fiscal Responsibility Act of 1982) is another attempt to limit the cost of medical care to the Federal government. It attempts to place limits on inpatient care costs, to limit the annual rate of cost increase for medical care, to provide incentives for reduction of costs, and to initiate prospective payment. All of these provisions developed as a result of the increase in Medicare and Medicaid costs.

### OTHER FORMS OF PRACTICES

Several means have been adopted to reduce the cost of medical care. We have mentioned the development of the HMO as a case in point. The response of the physician has been to create a prepaid medical practice but the evidence is not clear that it can compete with the HMO. Practice of medicine in clinics and in group practice is not cheaper than fee for service and may, in fact, be much higher depending upon the referrals among colleagues.

Enthoven (1980) has proposed that the entire system be scrapped in favor of a consumer choice proposal. His Consumer Choice Health Plan (CCHP) in the simplest form is a system which provides consumers with a finite expendable health care insurance fund and allows them to draw upon it for medical care as they see fit. The theory is good: it presupposes that the patient will choose the cheapest form of care if the quality is the same and that the patient will shop around for the best care. It also presupposes that physicians will compete for the best care at the cheapest price, as will hospitals and other parts of the system, so that the consumer will end up as a winner of added benefits. Homer (1982) has pointed out that this is not necessarily true. He gives data to indicate that in documented cases in Minnesota almost twice as many patients went to the hospital where the charges for a given operation were $4,587 than went to a hospital which charged $1,108 for the same service with the same apparent mortality and type of service. Other such cases can be documented. This suggests that other factors than costs may influence consumer decisions. However, the consumer is normally covered by insurance and with a finite sum of money for care the choices might be different.

Enthoven's proposal for CCHP is based upon a series of premises which may not be viable. In order for a patient choice system to control the health care delivery, it is essential that the patient have *multiple choice.* Several systems must be available from which patients can choose intensive, high volume, expensive care, or low volume, less intensive care, and pay accordingly. It is possible, for example, that groups of young, healthy individuals could opt for a system which had high deductibles, few benefits, and extremely low costs while the elderly might well opt for the opposite situation and pay accordingly. Regardless of the choice the *payment would be fixed.* The company or the government would issue vouchers for a fixed premium and the user would pay a deductible or co-insurance depending upon the kind of service desired. In order for such a system to work it would be necessary to have *open enrollment* so that anyone could enroll in the plan which suited that individual best and so that a choice of plans could be provided. The plans would have to be *community rated* in terms of the benefits and costs for the population to be served and finally all plans would have to guarantee a *standard benefit package* in order to assure that everyone was minimally covered. Enthoven (1980) believes that this will require the development of ADS (Alternate Delivery Systems) to provide the choices. The plan differs from the HMO in that everyone can choose the level of care within limits. Many economists believe that the plan will not work (Homer, 1982) because the consumer may choose other options than the best care at the cheapest price. In fact, as we have remarked, the consumer puts convenience, location, and perhaps other factors before price in considering health care options.

A method now under study for control of medical care is the creation of algorithms of treatment in which a scheme of logic, often computer driven, is used to define the problem and suggest treatment. The scheme developed in these cases is not designed to provide a cheaper medical treatment but to provide better decision making. One can argue that better decision making will eventually result in better and cheaper care but the evidence is not clear in this regard. On the other hand, the algorithm has been developed to allow nurse practitioners to treat patients under the supervision of physicians. In many cases, the method has proven to be cost effective. The system developed by the Army using Amosists (technicians performing the services) (Brown, 1978) has resulted in substantial reduction in costs of treatment, waiting times, and dissatisfaction. Wheeler (1983) claimed that the costs of pediatric practice could be reduced 15 percent with a proper algorithm with provision of equal and perhaps better care. Orient (1983) found that the number of prescriptions could be reduced about 40 percent if an algorithm was used in place of the usual diagnostic scheme and treatment.

In most cases, the algorithm developed has three major parts. The logic system provides a decision tree along which the practitioner can move in making a diagnosis. It usually contains a checklist to make sure that all events are covered in handling the patient, and finally it must include an audit of results and treatment in order to measure outcomes which are after all the final arbiter of practice.

Most algorithms are based on what amounts to a simple series of questions. These may be condensed to:

> What is the problem?
>
> Why is it important?
>
> What information is necessary to assess the scope of the problem?
>
> What are the criteria for measurement of the extent of the problem?
>
> How do the data compare with objective criteria?
>
> What are the deficiencies between the data and the objective criteria?
>
> What actions will correct the deficiency?
>
> What documentation is necessary?
>
> When does the problem need reassessment?
>
> What is the final conclusion?

Although there have been major advances in computer assisted diagnosis and in other medical applications, major hitches still exist in the systems. There are two major categories of approach: searching in a space for an answer in the most efficient manner and narrowing the search to smaller sets of data. These systems have been called "expert searches" by Gavater (1983). The development has moved from empirical associations in which a symptom is related to a disease to the functional relationships which exist in the system and can be pulled together to make a diagnosis. Because the expert must extract the information from the data set to be placed in the system, many of the systems tend to be broad but shallow or to be very narrow and restrictive. Until we can produce a system which combines the best features of both approaches, the average physician is likely to be unhappy with computer driven diagnosis. The development can be best demonstrated by the system developed by Dr. Jack Myers at Pittsburgh. The *Internist* program identifies some 500 diseases but suffers from the inability to make a general overview of a complicated problem and inadequate representation of the causes of disease. The newer system at Pittsburgh, *Caduceus,* can synthesize these elements and thus reach more explicit conclusions than previous systems.

We can summarize the types of organizations which are arising as a result of the costs of medical care. They can be listed as follows:

Private practice
Private group practice
Independent Physician Associations
Preferred Provider-Organizer
Health Maintenance Organization

These are listed in the order of decreasing costs and increasing control of costs. The only likely organization to succeed in reducing costs is one which deals in some form of prospective payment (PPO, HMO).

To the organizational structures of the physicians we can list the methods of payment as a means of controlling the system.

Retrospective Payment
Fixed Rate Payment
Prospective Payment
Diagnostic Related Group System
National Health Insurance
Consumer Choice(?)

Again the series is arranged in the order of increasing control of the system.

Still other approaches might well include:

Less Duplication of Facilities
Minimizing the Cost of Treatment
Increasing Physician Productivity
Prevention Education
Use of Generic Drugs
New Methods of Health Care
Competition
More Consumer Choice

Some interest is now being expressed in TRGs (Treatment Related Groups), which take into account not only the diagnosis but the cost of treatment as an overall package for reimbursement.

Another alternative was proposed some years ago by Barzel (1968), who proposed to examine the *expected* costs of treatment which might take into account preventive measures rather than the actual treatment costs as proposed above and thus force more prevention into the medical system. Still other methods of cost control have been advocated and some have been adopted in one form or another. Among the choices have been the institution of deductibles, which requires prepayment of a fixed amount by the consumer before the insurance company will pay additional costs, or the use of copayment in which the insured pays a fixed percentage of the costs which may be limited in either amount or type of service. Recent proposals to counter National Health Insurance have proposed the establishment of a catastrophic insurance which would pay medical costs exceeding a definite amount. Each of these measures has been suggested as means of reducing costs of care and making the consumer aware of costs. Obviously, the system of payment could be linked to any of the other parameters listed above.

An interesting relationship exists between the physician and the coverage for hospital care through insurance. If insurance pays for the hospital but not for physicians, when patients become ill they tend to seek hospital care. On the other hand, if both are covered, the cost is actually *less* than for hospital coverage alone since the patient can be reimbursed for the less expensive office call.

Another element which has been mentioned but which must also be considered in the context mentioned above is the method of determining the cost of insurance. The most common method now by the government is the community rating of reasonable fees for the area. We have already pointed out that this is a poor method in that services of the same quality and quantity may vary by 300 percent from one section of the country to another or from one part of a state to another part of the same state. Any rating should be based on a national average and the high-priced regions should be forced to adjust fees accordingly.

*Chapter 5*

# THE PHYSICIAN AND THE MILIEU

With the exception of those few physicians who practice in private offices and treat the nondebilitating diseases such as the allergies, most physicians are required to have available an armamentarium of apparatus and equipment which can be found only in the clinical laboratory or the hospital. The surgeon requires an immense supply of equipment and support systems. In addition, the patient is often treated in intensive care units of various kinds and with a variety of services such as inhalation therapy which can be administered only in an institution set up for the purpose. Most of these services are concentrated in the hospital. We are beginning to see the development of out-of hospital services such as emergency clinics, same-day surgeries, and dialysis centers but these are relatively few in number at the present time, and a very large part of physicians' time and effort is devoted to care of their patients in the hospital.

Physicians are trained from the time they are medical students to render tertiary care in a hospital setting. Perhaps 85 percent of their training in medical school is devoted to this end, and they are accustomed to the equipment and the services rendered. In addition, most physicians find it more comfortable to place patients in the hospital where they are readily available and concentrated in one area. That this may not be to the patients' advantage does not occur to the doctor.

The hospital is for the convenience of the physicians and they make the most of it. There is a great deal of pride in having "peeked, poked, prodded, and joked" with patient before 7:30 a.m. (Kramer 1982). The fact that patients are ill, may have had a bad night, and usually sleep until 8:00 a.m. does not alter the fact that they will be wakened at 6:00 a.m., bathed, and fed, and prepared for the doctor at 7:00 a.m. The scheduling of services is another case in point. It is for the doctor's convenience, not the patient's, that the x-ray department lines halls with prospective clients for hours before they are to be viewed and that surgical preparation often occurs many hours before the procedure. None of this is necessary. Simple queue theory would allocate resources and people so that patients could be scheduled at the time or close to the time that they are to be handled.

The hospital schedule is a masterful coordination of the desires of the workers. Patients are fed or dosed at the whims of the nurses' shifts. Patients are treated between office calls of the physician, and at no time is the patient considered.

In another respect, the hospital is the most costly hotel room in town. For prices ranging upward of $200 a day the patient is often treated to poor meals, poor service and a few aspirin. The argument can be made that services are available if necessary but the individual patient who does not need them should be discharged.

The hospital is a dangerous place to be. It has been estimated that 10 percent of the patients come out of the hospital in poorer condition than they went into it. Ten percent of the patients have some form of drug reaction, often because two incompatible drugs were given together. Patients are shocked by poor electrical connections, fall out of bed, slip on polished floors, and suffer myriad other mishaps due directly to the hospital and its method of operation. The situation is so prevalent that there is a disease entity called "iatrogenic" disease or disease caused by the treatment.

## The Hospital as a Business

Voluntary hospitals are not-for-profit institutions. This does not mean the hospital loses money. Frequently the hospital which is a part of a county health system does lose money because it is forced to take the indigent patient. But most voluntary hospitals are not in this situation. Such institutions manage to buy expensive equipment, build wings, open new services, and redecorate with the "non" profits which they receive. A hospital operates on the cost-plus basis. The total costs and the total receipts are balanced by the changing charges which are assessed. The very fact that hospital corporations which operate a series of hospitals can make about 12 percent profit each year indicates the slack in the system. Many large hospitals are now buying up small hospitals in the surrounding area in order to assure a flow of tertiary patients. This is not altruism. It is simply good business. The services also vary with the hospital. There are repeated complaints that patients are given unnecessary treatment and surgery depending upon their ability to pay, and that beds are kept full in order to maintain income. Of course, this requires the cooperation of the physicians, but in the final analysis their hospital privileges are granted by the hospital and they can be evicted if absolutely necessary. Most physicians find it advisable to cooperate.

Hospitals operate on a "keeping up with the neighbors" policy. If the hospital across the street gets a new piece of apparatus, it may attract more physicians or patients and it behooves the competition rapidly to obtain the equipment. The establishment of an open heart surgery unit in a hospital will lead to the establishment of such units in other hospitals in the area within a short time. The same principle applies to CAT scanners, PET scanners, and clinical laboratories.

Such developments may be harmful to the patient. As we have mentioned, when not enough surgery is done, the mortality rises and the patient is endangered.

The hospital must maintain income to pay staff and to function. This requires a bed census as high as possible. The average hospital requires an occupancy of about 85 percent to break even and the average hospital in this country is now about 75 percent occupied. This results in extreme pressure to admit patients and to keep patients in the hospital when they can more easily and more safely be discharged. It has been estimated that 25 percent of patients in a hospital are kept longer than necessary. In Great Britain where there are about one-half the hospital beds per unit of population, the estimates are that 30 percent of the patients could be released earlier with adequate home care (Carels, 1981) or not admitted in the first place. Many hospitals operate chains of small hospitals or helicopters (Life Flight) in order to fill beds and for the advertising provided by the size and visibility.

Several solutions have been proposed to the problems outlined above. One of the major trials has been the technique of Utilization Review. This technique identifies the patient and the treatment, assigns a definite period of stay, and maintains surveillance on activity. The procedures should result in fewer days of stay for the average patient, the elimination of patients who should not be in the hospital in the first place, and the determination of a standard of treatment. The procedure works well when the hospital is full but is less satisfactory when the hospital is partly empty and there is pressure to fill beds.

UR is the physicians' responsibility. They must agree to a standard of care for each disease which will be applied, must determine the hospital stay, and must be prepared to review the case of colleagues. This is a difficult task and not often carried out well. Censoring the physician who does not keep to the norms of the profession is rarely undertaken.

## HOSPITAL SERVICES AND THE PHYSICIAN

It has been remarked several times in the course of this book that regardless of the services provided by a hospital, none will be delivered without a physician order. On the other hand, the hospital can encourage such orders directly or indirectly. The purchase of large scale equipment and high technology is a direct incentive to use. Failure to keep beds filled is an indirect incentive. Pressure can be placed on the physicians to do more operations, to admit more patients, and to keep them in the hospital longer. This may be an advantage to the hospital.

**Table 4   The Relative Influences of Various Factors on the Rising Costs of Hospital Care Above the General Increase in the CPI**

| Major Influences | General Influences | Minor Influences |
|---|---|---|
| Number of Workers/bed | CPI increase | Wage Increases |
| Nonlabor Inputs (Technology) | Demands for More Care (aged, etc.) | Service Demands (General Population) |
| Third Party Payment | | |
| Overexpansion (Too Many Beds) | | |

The major return to a hospital in terms of charges occurs in the first few days of admission when lab tests are ordered, x-rays are taken, etc. After the procedures are completed, the hospital may become a hotel for the patient upon which little money is made because the costs of the bed and a diet approaches the charges. However, the beds are kept full and the empty bed costs the hospital about 75 percent of the financial costs of an occupied one. Hospitals look for charges.

The development of a wide variety of expensive services with the advent of high technology has made certain sections of the hospital a highly profitable enterprise. Pathology and the clinical laboratory attached to it, radiology and the new scanners, inhalation therapy, and the pharmacy are all highly profitable while the actual costs of dietary facilities and bed maintenance may be loss leaders.

It behooves us to look with some care at the services provided and the possibility of reducing costs in these high tech areas through physician control (Table 4).

## THE CLINICAL LABORATORY

The clinical laboratory is an entity which has both good and bad features as do most areas of hospital function. The number of tests has increased dramatically from 60 or so 30 years ago to several hundred which can be ordered and produced on demand. The complexity has developed from simple chemical tests for protein, fats, and carbohydrates to sophisticated enzyme assays, radioisotope tests, and genetic screening.

The clinical laboratories do perhaps 6 billion tests per year at a cost of about $20 billion dollars. Although tests are conducted in some 14,000 labs over the country, a large proportion are performed in the hospital lab. Many of the tests are now automated and some 12 to 20 different tests can be performed by machine on a single sample of blood or urine. The SMA-12 (the usual designation) is capable of running hundreds or thousands of tests per day on a routine basis. Yet problems remain.

Estimates by the Center for Disease Control, charged with the responsibility of determining quality of laboratory tests for the Federal government, indicate that 25 percent of all tests may be inaccurate. This occurs for several reasons. Samples are inadvertently mixed. Samples are lost, technicians err, or machines malfunction. Much of the error is due to human fallibility (Kennedy, 1975). Diagnostic kits are made by a variety of manufacturers for testing for various components of the blood or urine. Tests at one time on 44 different kits revealed that 32 were unsatisfactory (loc. cit.).

Sussman (1981) has reported that 33 percent of all "stat" orders, which means the test must be done immediately at extra cost to the patient, are totally unnecessary and are done on patients who may actually be normal.

The major failure in the system is the lack of understanding on the part of physicians and students. Medical students and residents order many more tests for the same disease than the practicing physician. The number of tests ordered by all MDs is indirectly related to the competence, experience, and past training of the physician. These facts can be clearly demonstrated. In studies where physicians were told of the cost of each test or where they were questioned as to the necessity for the test, the number of tests ordered decreased by up to 30 percent (Applegate, 1983; Daniels, 1973). Carels (1980) reported that many physicians order an electrolyte profile instead of an equally diagnostic serum potassium at much less cost.

Furthermore, when tests were performed on an outpatient

basis rather than on inpatients before a procedure, the cost dropped from $1,200 to $250 per patient (Blair, 1981). We have already mentioned the study of Connelly (1982) who found that for the same degree of severity and the same recovery rate, the number of tests increased by more than 100 percent in 7 years. Dixon (1974) found that a simple requirement for consultation before ordering tests considerably reduced the number ordered. Probably a main reason for the large number of tests is threefold. In the first place the physician has no idea of the costs of care (Long, 1983) and when informed of the large costs, revises the estimates. Secondly, it is simple and the hospital forms are devised to permit checking off a battery of requested tests instead of the one test required to confirm a diagnosis. The laboratory attempts to increase the volume of tests and income by providing order blanks for the wards which list most tests by battery (in conjunction with other tests) to encourage ordering in this fashion (Paris, 1976). The medical student and the resident are taught the procedure and uses of the battery. Thirdly, it is easier to depend upon technology to find a solution than to attempt a diagnosis based on reasoning. This is particularly distressing when so many tests are in error and when so few tests are actually used in the diagnosis. It has been reliably estimated that when a battery of tests is run the physician looks at perhaps 5 percent of the values and discards the remainder. It can be argued that the additional tests may reveal unsuspected disease but again the evidence indicates that the test results are rarely examined for this purpose and threat of disease is more often missed than revealed by the mass of data. In fact, Williams (1982) claims that tests are ordered because of inexperience, habit, pressure from the hospital, or to substitute for judgment.

A great many studies have been conducted on methods to decrease lab use. Proposals have been made to review orders before execution, to charge doctors for unnecessary tests, to provide education and feedback on need for tests, etc. It is interesting to note that when informed of costs of tests the average physician will reduce orders immediately as much as 30 percent. Unless there is constant reminder, however, the physician returns to habitual ordering patterns within a few months. One suggestion to counter this trend is to publish the orders of each physician for particular diseases. (Griner, 1872; Applegate, 1983; Cummings, 1982; Daniels, 1977).

## THE INTENSIVE CARE UNIT

Large metropolitan hospitals often have as many as 10 intensive care units utilizing about 25 percent of the hospitals resources for about 5 percent of the patients. The average cost can easily exceed $1,000 per day. The question under discussion is not whether intensive care units should be available but whether they are unwisely used. Intensive care units are expensive to maintain, skilled personnel must be available at all times, expensive equipment is required, and supplies are many and varied. A hospital must attempt to keep the unit as full as possible in order to make a return on the large investment. As a result, the units are often overused for cases which should not have been placed in intensive care in the first place. Secondly, here again hospitals suffer from "keeping up with the Joneses" syndrome. Every hospital feels that it is essential to have at least one and perhaps several intensive care units in order to compete in service with neighboring institutions.

A study of intensive care units in Massachusetts a few years ago (Bloom, 1974) revealed that the state had 336 beds in ICUs and the maximum which could be used at any one time was about 250. The excess beds raised the costs for the users of the occupied beds without contributing to medical care. There is also considerable doubt about the effectiveness of many intensive care units. The most money and the most time are invested in those patients who die, and not in those who live. The average cost for a stay in intensive care was $14,000 (Collen, 1976) in 1976 and may be double that now. Of this cost 83 percent was expended on nonsurvivors. This raises the question of choice of patients. Should a patient who is unlikely to survive be placed in intensive care or should the care be devoted to those who have a chance of living?

There is evidence that many patients are placed in intensive care for no good reason. It may be simpler to check on a condition or to monitor signs with the equipment in intensive care but that is no reason to use an expensive facility. Knaus (1981) found that 86 percent of patients admitted to an ICU required nothing but monitoring and had no active treatment at all. These studies suggest that ICU patients can be divided into three types. About 50 percent of the patients should never have been admitted to the unit and would have done equally well on the wards, about 30 percent of the patients had a 30 percent mortality and probably benefited from the treatment, and the rest of the patients had much higher mortalities and probably did not benefit and perhaps should not have been admitted.

Furthermore, the ICU is lavish in the use of laboratory tests and extracorporeal devices. There are many who claim that some of the tests are really necessary, and serve to provide diagnosis and treatment, and the rest are in fact window-dressing. Myers (1981) found that only about 5 percent of the laboratory tests are actually used in formulating treatment. In addition, the excess of extracorporeal devices for which the need is not clear cut has often resulted in iatrogenic disease from clots, poor circulation, restricted movements, wrong administration of solutions, and myriad other problems which are compounded in the ICU because of the massive volume of services provided.

With this general survey of the problem we can consider the special ICUs which abound. Almost every hospital of any size has a cardiac ICU to monitor the heart patients. There is considerable question as to the efficiency of these units. In the first place, as mentioned above, it is expensive and fruitless to pay ICU rates for simple monitoring when nothing else is being done for the patient. Yet this is the function of many ICUs. Secondly, the evidence from England indicated that cardiac patients actually do better when sent home than when they are kept in an ICU. Abel Smith (1976) and Bloom (1973) have calculated that the costs far outweigh the benefits of coronary care units.

The perinatal ICU is another form of intensive care unit for the premature infant. There is no question but that the ICU does save the lives of many premature infants who would otherwise have died. The problem here is the living—not the dying. Boyle (1983) has estimated that premature infants saved will cost society for the rest of their lives in that most such babies suffer from a variety of defects which will later result in medical costs. In addition, many dollars are spent on infants who die after intensive treatment. Attempts at sustaining life in such individuals should be viewed with caution. A classic example are the *spina bifida* children, many of whom are saved through pediatric surgery and ICUs. These infants never have a reasonable quality of life, require intensive care, life-long expense, and most do not live more than a few years and there is considerable question as to the value to society of an ICU to maintain such a clinical anomaly.

Pascarelli (1982) points out that as a result of the establishment of intensive care for postnatal patients we have increased the demand for ambulatory services for learning disabilities, mental retardation, chronic illness, allergies, drug addiction, and nutritional deficits. And, of course, we do not yet know the effect on future generations if such infants grow up to reproduce.

Another intensive care problem is the prenatal mother who now receives fetal monitoring as a routine matter before and during delivery. Fetal monitoring units cost about $25,000 each and most hospitals are now equipped with them. The evidence suggests that perhaps 90 percent of them are unneeded (Haverkamp, 1979). Haverkamp estimates that $80 million per year is wasted in totally unnecessary fetal monitoring.

The same statements can be made about renal disease. The number of patient with ESRD (end stage renal disease) is increasing more than 10 percent per year. As we have remarked, a number of patients on dialysis were originally supposed to receive renal transplants and the dialysis was a stopgap measure. However, the number of available kidneys is small and the number of rejections is high (about 60 percent for nonsibling kidneys). The 5-year survival is about 40 percent for nonrelated kidney donations. The kidney patient on dialysis has an expected life of 9 years at a cost of about $300,000 or more.

Another fad which has arisen in the hospital is the use of inhalation therapy. Inhalation therapy is useful for some respiratory disorders but the evidence is mounting that it may be dangerous to many patients (Gibson, 1974). Yet every hospital has a unit, and the units are heavily used.

A recent report by the OTA (Schleffler, 1981) suggests that

although respiratory therapy has had a wide popularity there is no clear demonstration that any method other than administration of oxygen for anoxia has any benefit. There is no evidence to document the effectiveness of IPPB (intermittent positive pressure breathing). Despite these obvious facts, about 30 percent of all patients receive some form of respiratory therapy. Fortunately, there is a real indication of decline in the use of IPPB but other forms of therapy which are not well documented are taking its place.

Many ICUs function as a geriatric deathbed. The old and dying are placed in intensive care when both the patient and the physician are aware that the treatment is futile. It would appear cruel to attach a variety of monitoring instruments to a dying patient to satisfy family or the self-protective sense of the physician.

The situation is difficult to correct. Utilization review should eliminate from an ICU those who should not be in one, and should limit the stay of those who are admitted; but as we have remarked before, such reviews are effective only when the beds are full. Many ICU beds should be closed permanently, or Medicaid and the insurance companies should refuse to pay for treatment in them unless it is fully documented.

## The Hospital and High Technology

The hospital has been in the forefront in the establishment of high-tech, high-cost centers for various services. Again, there is an ambiguity in such developments. On the one hand, many of the techniques are invaluable, have saved lives, and have been of cost benefit to medicine. On the other hand, most of them have been exploited through overuse, put to purposes for which they were not intended, and are in oversupply. The classic example is the CAT scanner. Computerized Axial Tomography (CAT) is an x-ray technique which essentially creates three-dimensional images of the body. It was devised in the first place to examine difficult-to-reach areas such as the head for invasive tumors or aneurysms. It was rapidly expanded to soft tissues and is now widely used to examine all parts of the body. Two problems have arisen. In the first place, the technique has been used where it is not suitable. When a diagnosis is 95 percent certain, it is a waste of time and money to confirm the other 5 percent with an expensive ($250) test. Yet many of the diagnoses made with the CAT scanner are backup to lab tests or other x-rays and have questionable value. Secondly, the "keeping up with the Joneses" syndrome again becomes apparent. When one hospital has a CAT scanner, others must also have theirs. Sweden and England have the same mortality for the common diseases and they use the CAT scanner (invented in England, by the way) about 50 percent as much as it is used in the United States. Those countries have determined that one CAT scanner per one million people is the correct ratio to keep the machine busy, have well-trained people to run it, and to use it for the proper examinations. In the U.S. we have, in some cities, as many as one scanner for 100,000 people. When a machine is expensive ($500,000) and requires expensive trained personnel to operate it two events must occur. The prices must be raised to pay for the machine, and the number of scans must be increased to utilize excess services available. Both methods are used extensively. We are now in a new generation of scanner, the PET (Positron Emmission Tomography) which is much more expensive because of the generating source and which may prove to be useful in only a few special cases. Again the PET scanner will be used to confirm diagnosis, but this is largely for the doctor's protection rather than for the good of the patient. NMR (Nuclear Magnetic Resonance) machines are now developed, and will be in hospitals soon for the future examination of the body. The same statements can again be repeated about the advantages and disadvantages of this machine.

We are continually faced with the problem of what to do with excess time and capability of expensive machines. The hospitals buy the machines partly at the instigation of the physician who is always intrigued with a new gadget but they fully expect to make a profit from their operation. Machines are usually purchased with the assurance that they can be kept busy. This may mean hiring new staff with clinical or research experience in such machines with the resultant cost to the patient who does not need or use the machine. Hospitals rarely use the cost-centered approach in which they determine the cost to operate and the income of each unit separately and then price services accordingly. Usually all costs are combined and this is divided into all income to determine a daily rate. Expensive machines simply raise the rate for everyone. Although this is an oversimplification, the requirement of a cost-centered approach would eliminate much technology, especially if use were restricted to actual need.

Another lucrative income area requiring high technology is the open heart surgical unit. About 200,000 bypass operations are done each year at a cost of about $15,000 in hospital charges. Bypass surgery is in considerable doubt as to its efficacy. Studies at the VA several years ago suggested that perhaps 50 percent or more of surgeries could be avoided with medical treatment, and a recent study of 1,200 consecutive bypass cases by Ralimtoola (1983) found that 23 percent had to be reoperated upon and 40 percent still had angina after the operation, while the rest had from good to fair improvement. This would appear to be a poor investment from the cost benefit viewpoint especially since it is likely that some of those could have been helped by drugs.

As we have mentioned there are many who believe that the community would be better served if all high technology were grouped in centers. There have been proposals to create heart surgery centers (Finklet, 1981) doing several hundred operations per year. There have also been proposals to place all CAT scanners in a single center and refer all patients to that location. There have been attempts to create a central laboratory for all chemical analysis. In principle the idea is a good one. The few examples in practice suggest that better regulation would be necessary before success could be assured. The private dialysis centers around the country are expensive and often mechanical in operation so that patients become rapidly depressed. A few laboratories which perform millions of analyses per year have been discredited by the CDC for poor performance. There are large centers for heart surgery such as the Texas Heart Institute but there is no sign they have reduced costs or diminished the number of patients treated.

The one attempt to regulate technology has been through the Certificate of Need Program (CON) in which requests for equipment above $100,000 are reviewed by a committee composed of members of the health community. These committees operated under the HSA (Health Services Agency) but with the demise of that unit, CON may well be on its way out. The system did not work well at its best. Trade-offs occurred regularly. It was easy for an administrator to say "You vote for my new x-ray and I'll vote for your CAT scanner." The committee was dominated by professionals both in number and in expertise and all too often their decisions were made on a quid pro quo basis. Tighter controls are necessary.

## Hospital Beds

A good (or bad?) example of the overbedding which occurs is in Houston. The city has 20,443 beds for about 2 million people or one bed per 100 people. A reasonable supply is considered to be one bed for 800 people. There is no wonder that Houston hospitals advertise their wares. As a result, 96 percent of the hospitals are multi-institutional arrangements and some 56 percent of the hospitals are for profit. Houston is obviously a lucrative market, aided by the large number of physicians practicing in the area, and the reputation of the Texas Medical Center. Hospitals in Houston make no bones about the fact that multi-institutional arrangements help in patient referral and keeping beds full. There is also no wonder that medical costs in Houston are increasing about 50 percent faster than in other parts of the country.

Harris (1975) found that 25 percent of all beds were unneeded and were kept filled on the basis of comfort, convenience to the physician, or safety, rather than medical need. This means that the public is paying $20 billion or about $100 more per person per year than is necessary for health costs.

Hospital stays are often of poor quality. Patients rank hospitals relatively low on quality of care (77 percent of all questioned patients) (McLachlan, 1976). Risks in hospitals are significant, as we have already mentioned. Drugs are mismanaged and too many drugs are administered (Lawson, 1976). As many as 20 drugs are administered to the same patient. There is little wonder that drug reactions are common.

Finally, half of all hospital stays are for surgery of one kind or another. Review of cases might reduce the number of operations. The second opinion was proposed and some statistics indicate it reduces operations 20 or so percent.

The above clearly indicates that the demand for beds is artificial. HMOs provide equal services to general practice tertiary care and use about one-half the hospital beds per unit of population (Harris, 1975). Yet hospitals are continually expanding and new ones are being built. Again the system is at fault. As we increase the supply of doctors, and the number of people who are insured, the demand for hospital beds increases. The institution of a copayment plan for hospital care would materially decrease usage, and the restriction on the number of beds in a community to a given number per unit of population would be effective in decreasing the number of new beds built each year. We are now spending about $7 billion per year on new facilities. The actual need may be for one-tenth of this amount.

The hospital has a wastage which would not be tolerated in any business. A business operated at 75 percent capacity would shut down lines of production and fire employees. The hospital takes the position that an emergency may arise today which would require the staff and beds, though this is extremely unlikely. Hospitals could adopt the industrial position and close wards and lay off employees rather than pad bed-census by keeping patients for longer periods of time.

The hospital operates with two administrative systems which would not be tolerated by any industry. On one hand, there is the administrator with a staff of lay personnel who manages the hospital and, on the other hand, there is the chief of staff with his or her professional group which manages the patient care. The two are often at odds. Because of the system, an enormous amount of paperwork must flow between units of the hospital. This is wasteful and inefficient.

One of the problems of productivity in hospitals is the poor relationship between managers and workers. The highly professional skills required of some of the personnel tends to denigrate the skills and work of the majority of the workers, many of whom must do menial work. The situation is worse in the medical profession and the hospital than in the factory, where recent surveys by the Public Agenda Forum of New York found that only 23 percent of workers found any correlation between their jobs and their pay; only 13 percent believed that hard work would be rewarded; 23 percent said that they did not contribute full effort to any job; and most claimed that the employer did not

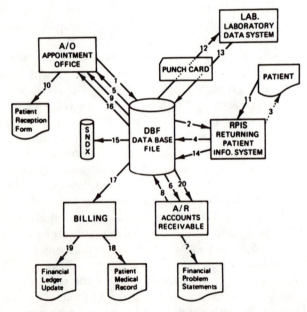

Computer-based data flow interrelating administrative systems. From Rockart (1973).

Figure 5. The interrelationships between elements in a large computer-based information system for the hospital (from Brown, J.H.U., & Dickson, J.F., *Advances in Biomedical Engineering* (Vol. 6), New York: Academic Press, 1976, by permission).

know how to motivate the workers. About two-thirds of all workers in the survey wanted pay for performance as the most desirable feature of any position. The report claims that managerial skills have not kept pace with changes in the workplace.

The operating base of the hospital is in the patient record, which will determine the costs of care, the type of care rendered, and the procedure conducted. Yet the record is often unavailable, not up to date, and poorly written. Hospitals need a patient record system which is tied to cost accounting, housekeeping, and patient care (Fig. 5). Several hospitals in England use microcomputers (Apple II) to perform many of these tasks and the El Camino Hospital outside San Francisco uses the computer to solve all of the record problems. There are almost no written records and the system is tied together so that all parts interrelate.

## The Physician and the Drug Industry

We are a nation of drug addicts. Last year (1981) physicians prescribed 650,000,000 doses of one form of medication or another. This does not take into account the untold billions of doses of over-the-counter (OTC) drugs taken for every sort of imagined or real ailment. The data indicate that the majority of drugs prescribed by physicians may be of doubtful benefit. The drugs most commonly dispensed were antihistaminics, antiallergens, antibiotics along with tranquilizers and sedatives (Koch, 1982). In addition, most of the drugs prescribed (75 percent) were by brand names despite the fact that generic drugs are equally potent and much cheaper. The use of generic drugs can be defended also on the basis that 70 percent of all prescriptions called for a drug with a single ingredient rather than a mixture or combination of drugs.

Overprescribing and the use of brand names in prescribing are due mainly to the promotional efforts of the drug companies. It has been estimated that the drug companies spend up to 25 percent of total operating costs in advertising (Abel-Smith, 1976). The advertising through mail, magazines, representatives, and sample distribution costs the drug companies about $5,000 per doctor per year. There is little question about the efficacy of the advertisements. Despite the obvious conflict of interest, the AMA has steadfastly refused to ban drug advertising from its journals.

Drug information is usually misleading. One needs only to recall the numerous incidents in the daily newspapers about the withdrawal of drugs from the market, the side effects of many drugs (thalidomide) and the suits brought against the drug companies. These tales or hearsay are often based on solid fact. The National Academy of Sciences reviewed the efficacy of trade-name drugs a few years ago. Of some 4,500 drug preparations reviewed, only 35 percent were determined to be efficacious and useful.

Pricing policy of the drug company leads to unproductive results. Berki (1977) has reported that some drug prices vary by 200 percent from one company to another for the same drug and that prices in a pharmacy for the same batch number of a drug may vary by 130 percent from week to week. On the international market the situation is worse. Librium as a trade-name drug can be produced for about $5/kg. It sells in the U.S. for about $20/kg and in some foreign countries for as much as $1,250/kg (Abel-Smith, 1976). In other situations the reverse is true. Estrogens, which are given in large quantities, are much cheaper in Europe. There is no detectable reason for the difference.

The administration of drugs is so common that almost every consultation with a physician results in a prescription. The average patient gets about five prescriptions per year. Coupled with the use of the drugs must be their preparation. At the present time, about 5 percent of drugs are compounded by the pharmacist. The remainder are prepared by the producing company and dispensed by the pharmacists under their label. This results in a double markup with no added gain to the patient.

The extent of the drug-related problem can be estimated by the fact that some 5 percent of all hospital admissions are due to drug-related problems and Jick (1976) and others have claimed that as many as 35 percent of all patients suffer some drug-related problem while in the hospital.

Unfortunately, the drug companies have created problems in other ways. The favorite method of selling drugs is to use the "detail man" who visits the physicians, presents samples and endeavors to persuade them to use the product. Many, if not most, of these sales representatives are untrained, simply repeat the company literature, and gloss over difficulties. Yet some 50 percent of physicians rely almost exclusively on these people for information on new drugs and on treatment regimes. The sales representative not only provides information but sways the physician with gifts and elaborate presentations. As a result, many doctors still use drugs whose efficacy is in great doubt. A classic case of misuse is chloroamphenicol which causes blood dyscrasias and death in patients and yet comprises about 1 percent of all antibiotic prescription in this country and as much as 5 percent abroad. Parenthetically, the drug company makes enough of this antibiotic to treat 2 illnesses per person/year although the estimated need is to treat one illness per person every 5 to 10 years.

The physician could adopt several simple steps to reduce drug costs to the patient. In the first place, the use of generic rather than name brand drugs would reduce drug costs about 25 percent. The banning of advertising in journals and barring the use of sales representatives would also reduce the cost and use of drugs considerably. The careful review of the use of drugs by PSO committees would halt improper use. For example, there are many cases of doctors who still administer penicillin for the common cold despite the clear evidence of ineffectiveness.

Secondly, the OTC market is enormous and is continuously expanding. The drug companies spend millions of dollars in TV advertising every year and with good effect. Smith (1972) found that 29 percent of the population get all of their drug information from the television. Children believe about 70 percent or more of the ads although review panels conclude that the advertisements are only about 30 percent correct. Almost no program provides adequate, factual information which can be used to make a logical choice.

The use of drugs by the public is exaggerated by the general hypochondria. It has been estimated that about 80 percent of most office visits are for trivial reasons and Lewis Thomas (1978) has remarked that most diseases will cure themselves if let alone. The hypochondria is assisted by the physician who prescribes vitamins or antihistamines for these patients.

We have mentioned the fact that the physician tends to order a great deal of drugs. The average office visit results in a prescription for two or more drugs. As mentioned, most of these drugs are proprietary when generic drugs would do as well. In the hospital drugs are administered ad libitum. Patients coming to the office usually expect to receive a prescription although more than 60 percent do not take the drugs when prescribed (Davis, 1966). The treatment of patients is not up to quality standards. A review of physicians' records and drugs ordered indicated that only 27 percent were treating hypertension correctly, only 33 percent were handling ulcers correctly, and only 11 percent could deal adequately with upper respiratory infection (Brook, 1975).

Of greater concern is the information that doctors tend to obtain a large part of their medical information from ads and other drug company information. The drug companies use several methods to assure sales. The advertising campaigns are among the largest in industry. Free journals are produced, free samples handed out, and "detail men" are constantly on the go visiting the physician with the latest drug information. Obviously, the information must be slanted. It is very unlikely that a Searle sales representative will recommend Upjohn products, and the doctor listens. Fifty-seven percent of all information on drugs comes from sales representatives, 27 percent from advertising and samples, and only 7 percent from the medical journals. With potent drugs physicians are a little more careful. When they prescribe such drugs, it is because of information obtained 25 percent from sales representatives, 30 percent from ads, and 20 percent from journals, and the rest from contact with fellow physicians. They tend to favor those sales representatives whom they know best and to use the product of the company they represent (Herman, 1976).

The strong contact between the drug and other technical industries lasts through life. It begins with the students' first day in medical school when they are given a bag of test instruments and drug samples and extends to the mature physician. In addition, some 15 percent of all physicians own pharmacies, drug supply houses, or the like, and this is a direct conflict of interest.

## DRUGS AND INFORMATION

The lack of information for the patient is a major complaint of the health care system. The physician aggravates this feeling. The patient is given drugs by brand name which tell nothing about the type of drug. Secondly, the physician often instructs the pharmacist not to give the patient the instructions sheet which accompanies any drug detailing the side effects. In many cases, the company does not inform the physician of all of the side effects. The FDA is now proposing that *government*-written pamphlets accompany potent drugs to explain to the physician and, it is hoped, the patient, the side effects to be expected. The drug companies are also proposing to advertise directly to the patient in addition to the long-time practice of advertising in professional journals. Again the physicians oppose such a trend on the ground that they will be besieged by patients for potent advertised drugs for specific conditions.

Problems with drugs have plagued physicians for decades. Oraflex was removed from the market after several deaths and the drug used to treat mild diabetes, Orinase, was discovered to have major side effects only after several years of use. Some accommodation between the physician using the drug and the company making it must be reached so that safe and useful drugs reach the market.

The situation is made worse by the fact that the physician often gives the wrong drug, the wrong dosage, or the wrong instructions. In one large hospital, 15 percent of all prescriptions were incorrectly written and 50 patients per day had to spend an average of 15 minutes each to get prescriptions checked and rewritten. The time taken up was spent largely by the pharmacist who had to check the drug or phone the doctor for instructions (Ingrim, 1983). Physicians write about $1 billion worth of prescriptions per year for sleeping pills and some 40 percent of all old people receive such a prescription despite the clear evidence that sleep apnea occurs in such individuals and is exacerbated by the drug (Kripke, 1983).

Other studies have indicated that antibiotics have been prescribed inappropriately about 40 percent of the time (Jewesson,

1983) and Walson (1981) reported that wrong prescriptions are particularly prevalent in pediatric clinics.

One means of control of the costs of drugs has been adopted by the Medicare. This concept is entitled the Maximum Allowable Costs (MAC) and sets a limit on the cost of drugs based on the manufacturer's price and prescriptions. The concept arose when it was found, for example, that propoxphene cost 4 cents to make and package and the average druggist charge was $3.18. The program is aimed at forcing the use of generic drugs and could conceivably save a great deal of money. There has been great opposition on the part of both druggists and physicians, the druggist because of the profit motive and the physicians because they are used to ordering drugs by the brand name as given them by the sales representatives, and ordering by the generic name requires more work in looking up names in formularies (Lee, 1983).

## AMBULATORY CARE

In an attempt to fill empty beds with inpatients, the hospitals have resorted to the establishment of ambulatory care clinics. The units are often located at remote sites to encourage neighborhood contacts and referrals. However, the clinics suffer from several difficulties.

In the first place, the establishment of an ambulatory care unit is often resented by the doctors in practice in the vicinity. In fact, the physicians are often a part of the hospital referral system and a clinic in direct competition may send their business to another location. Secondly, the clinics are more expensive than either the practitioner or the stand-alone clinic. The excuse is that the hospital has ongoing indirect costs which must be borne by the outpatients as well as the inpatients, and that the hospital provides all of the services needed for any case which may arise. As we have mentioned, the number of cases which come to an ambulatory clinic (emergency department) may have less that 10 percent emergencies and the rest can be handled easily with routine practice. The number coming to an ambulatory clinic for emergency must be much less than that number; so the argument of resources which must be provided does not hold up.

Hospital-based ambulatory care units have several characteristics in common. They include:

A coordinated center of care
A separate physical unit
Reduced waiting time
Full-time professional staff
Assigned residents
Sophisticated financial arrangements

Some of the reasons they have not been uniformly successful include:

Large numbers of low-income patients
Inefficiency
Greater specialty care than GP, therefore greater costs
Outpatients may help pay for educational cost of house staff
Usually viewed by hospital as an inpatient care system input rather than a stand-alone unit
Allocation of indirect costs which should not be included in outpatient service (Pascarelli, 1982)

As we have mentioned, many hospitals are turning to community-based clinics for referrals. There are now about 1,000 in the country. They serve to attract providers to underserved areas, to capture a local patient population, and to help provide program integration. Moreover, these clinics provide for the elderly. In Chelsea Village, New York City, the cost of providing community health and home health care dropped the cost per person from $2,100 per month in a nursing home to $850 per month including all medical care (Brickner, 1978).

Ambulatory outpatient departments face several liability situations which must be handled with care. Medical malpractice must be carefully controlled. It is harder to control malpractice when the patient is walk-in and leaves without resolution of the problem. If the patient does not obey the order given by the physicians, he or she may have an adverse condition and sue. The unit also faces the problem of when to treat or not to treat a patient. Many apparent diseases are psychosomatic (estimates run as high as 80 percent) and the time and funds of the outpatient department are taken up by these individuals. The outpatient facility also faces the problem of failure to treat the patient properly and promptly and to handle the injury which may result from long waiting times or incorrect treatment by staff. Finally, the problem of liability arises on every hand. Much of the liability is shared—the unit and the physician are both to blame because the unit failed to prevent a physician from performing an improper treatment. Vicarious responsibility arises when the employee of the unit does something incorrect to the patient and the clinic is responsible for that action. The clinic is also responsible for treatment which is rendered after a delay, treatment which is offered over the phone, and for failure to triage emergency patients promptly. Each of these problems increases the need for supervision, and may increase costs.

On the other hand, patients must be helped. They come to the clinic because they have no physician, they are unable to find the family doctor, or they have been referred by the physician (in an emergency).

Hospitals have other reasons for setting up ambulatory care centers. These can be listed:

They provide increased revenue

They provide revenue for hospital services (x-ray, lab, etc.)

They increase efficiency by using facilities which are not fully utilized

They enhance the reputation of the hospital

Finally, they provide a service which is needed

Most hospital outpatient departments offer lip service to prevention but this is absolutely not in their best interests. However, at least one group has attempted to make prevention a part of the conventional medical practice in a positive manner. The INSURE project described by Logson (1983) charges a fee to patients for prevention. For this fee they receive examinations, consultations, and briefings on prevention. The cost has been about $35 per year per patient but the author estimates the cost benefit as much greater than this sum. A survey of patients indicated that they were willing to pay a reasonable amount for prevention if they could be assured of active attention by the staff.

## MEDICAL INSURANCE

The payers of the system, the insurance companies which now cover about 85 percent of the population, receive bills from the physician, pay them, and bill the patient for cost plus overhead. Despite claims to the contrary, there is little effort to control costs because the insurance company has little incentive to do so. Finally, the patient receives services often without understanding the service or the costs or without even seeing the bill except for the yearly premium from the insurance company.

It is obvious that an open-loop system exists. The only way to close the loop is to make the patient a part of the feedback system. There are two ways to close the loop. One method is to educate patients to costs of care, alternative methods, etc., so that they can pressure insurance companies, physicians, and hospitals for information, and the Federal government for regulation. A second method is to make consumers to some degree their own provider so that they can help to reduce costs in the system. Experiments are now under way in the hope that an adequate feedback can be established.

## POSSIBLE CONTROLS

We have already remarked on the possibility of reducing costs by walk-in clinics and ambulatory surgery. Many other cost-saving measures can be adopted with loss of revenue to the hospital but increased efficiency of service and reduced costs to the patient.

Some heart surgery centers have now proposed that the patient come in the day before surgery to obtain blood typing, and other laboratory tests before surgery. The cost is about $250 rather than $1,000 if the tests are performed in house (Balir, 1981).

Many of the procedures for which the patient is admitted and kept overnight in the hospital can be performed easily on an outpatient basis. Patients can be admitted later and discharged earlier.

A major part of the cost of the hospital is the overuse of services. There is a clear correlation between the availability of services and their use (Bohr, 1980). As soon as a hospital provides the equipment for open heart surgery, more of such surgery is done although the survival rates may not be satisfactory. New services should be carefully questioned.

The use of highly specialized equipment is a function of where it is found. Documentation makes it clear that those physicians who have x-ray machines in their offices use (the machine) more than those physicians who must refer the patient to a radiologist. It is not unusual for the hospital to perform an ECG and the physician to charge an extra fee for reading it, even though a cardiologist is available. If a patient is placed in a high tech situation (ICU) the physician charges more per visit than if the patient were placed on a ward. The assignment of patients to a series of tests may not benefit physicians directly through "kickbacks" but it does benefit them in that they have released their own time for further income-producing efforts. The use of technology is also complicated by the fact that most physicians tend to use one method of treatment even when another has been shown to be more effective or the adopted one has been demonstrated to be less effective. Each behaves as if his or her method was the only method and no gray area existed (Wennberg, 1980).

Furthermore, the conflict of interest extends over a broad range of often almost undefinable areas. The CON boards required by law in communities are a good example. The professionals are often in a heavy majority in actual numbers or in knowledge and as a result can influence decisions on construction, purchase of equipment, etc. It is difficult to imagine decisions which would conflict with the physicians' best interests being adopted by such boards.

Hospital days can be easily restricted. Bognanni (1982) states that a 14 percent reduction in hospital days can be obtained immediately by stricter allocation of beds. In another experience, the HMO's in the country have an average of 418 hospital days/ 10,000 people, while an average population has 919 days for the same number of people. It can be claimed that the HMO selects its population but other restrictive measures have produced the same downward trend in occupancy.

In another view, Kaluzny (1976) has examined the problem of organizational "slack," which he defines as the ratio of assistants and associates on the staff divided by the patient days. He points out that up to a point this is a good thing because it permits the opportunity to think and innovate but beyond that point it becomes a liability in terms of costs. The increase in the number of workers for the care of each patient has increased from about 1.5 to more than 3.0 within the last few years and with little evidence of decreasing mortality from increasing use of technology. Questions can be raised about the need for increased staff.

There have been several suggestions (Wood, 1982) that hospital charges be based on services. In other words, the charge for a bed would be not uniform but would depend upon the nursing care demanded and the other services which the hospital must provide. If an individual was occupying a bed with no services required other than meals, or was partly ambulatory, the charges would be minimal. It has also been proposed that the same system be applied to the physician. The average Medicaid charge for a visit is $16 regardless of the treatment or the length of time the patient spends with the doctor. In so-called "Medicaid Mills" the time spent may be about 6 minutes per patient (Mitchell, 1980).

Relating charges to services would materially change the billing system in health care. Physicians oppose the proposal adamantly. Charging each patient a different rate would be a major bookkeeping problem and the ability of the government to check on actual services and charges would be minimal.

Caterinicchio (1983) tried to determine a more exact cost by allocating nurse services on the basis of need with a computer model. At the present time the nurse charges, which are a large part of the hospital bill, are charged on a per diem basis (Fig 4). If the charges are based on actual use of nurses by the patient the average charges drop markedly and considerable reductions in hospital costs can be obtained. When the hospital and the physician work together to assign nursing duties as actually needed, the costs might be reduced further.

Another point of contention between hospitals and physicians lies in the provision of services. Tatchell (1983) and others have pointed out that hospitals operate on one of two methods. In one method the hospital provides all the services which it believes to be necessary or which the doctor demands, and "markets" its service in order to be sure they are used effectively even though expensively. In the second type, the hospital provides the services based on the needs of the community without consideration of the marketing aspect. This is the system used to some degree in Sweden and England where CAT scanners and other equipment are allocated on the basis of population rather than hospital desires (Tatchell, 1983). In the United States the hospitals compete with each other for equipment so that all hospitals have relatively the same ability to deliver services from the standpoint of equipment if not personnel. Evidence is clear that various hospitals have different mixes of patients depending upon location, patient income, and physicians in attendance, and equipment and services should be based on this factor. Grouping of cases into DRGs (Diagnostic Related Grouping) (Fetter, 1980) and providing services based on these categories may reduce costs substantially. However, in the ultimate, the physician is the final arbiter and if he demands the service it will be provided.

In some hospitals, a revolution has been under way. In Memphis, if a nurse or aide fails to respond to a call bell within 1 minute, $10 is deducted from the daily bed charge. If the room is not taken care of promptly and well, another $10 is deducted from the charges. At a hospital in Las Vegas every patient is seen within 1 minute of entering regardless of the degree of emergency. These are all for-profit hospitals. The majority of hospitals are voluntary hospitals with little concern for these mundane problems.

The for-profit motive may not be all bad. AMI (American Medical International) has a group of CAT scanners which can be leased on demand to individual hospitals thus saving the cost of purchase of a unit at every hospital. Most of the for-profit hospitals are newer, better equipped, and more efficient than the average voluntary hospital, which is about 25 years old. In addition, the for-profit hospitals paid about $450 million in taxes in 1981 while the voluntary hospitals drew on the tax dollar. The comparisons are obvious.

Boards of voluntary hospitals and their staffs complain that for-profit hospitals skimp on services in order to make profits. The for-profits counter that their profit comes from more efficient operation as opposed to poorer service and point out also that questionnaires have revealed that patients appear to be well satisfied with the standard of care.

We have remarked that hospitals typically operate at about 75 percent of capacity and that this places a strain on the hospital finances and on the physician, who is often under pressure to fill beds. MacStravick (1981) proposed a solution to both problems. He suggested that hospital admissions could be governed by several new approaches. In one model, a patient would be admitted under three protocols: emergency cases would be admitted at once, scheduled patients would be admitted on a prior determined schedule, and call-in patients would be admitted when space permitted. Obviously, doctors would be forced to follow the protocol and admit their patients under demand rather than at their doctors' convenience. Secondly, a protocol could be set up on a capacity basis where patients would be admitted to the emptiest hospital which had the facilities to provide the necessary service. Again, both hospitals and physicians would have to agree to allow the physician to practice in various hospitals and the physician would have to sacrifice the convenience of operating in a single hospital to the total advantage of the system. Unfortunately, neither is likely to happen in the foreseeable future. It should also be noted that patients are likely to be dissatisfied with the system because many prefer the hospital nearest to their homes or the hospital which has the best reputation in their eyes.

## CONTROL IN THE HOSPITAL

As physicians learn more about the technology which is available they may rely less upon the high tech diagnostic instrumentation and more upon the assist devices which aid in their thinking and ability to make an accurate diagnosis. Dr. Jack Myers at Pittsburgh has long been an advocate of computer controlled diagnosis. Programs are already available or in the development phase for drug treatment programs, cancer treatment, and drug compatibility. The idea really began with Lawrence Weed at Vermont about 20 years ago but has expanded rapidly. The leaders have been the Stanford Program, a program at Massachusetts General Hospital under Dr. Octo Barnett, the program in Salt Lake City under Dr. Homer Warner, the program at Washington University in St. Louis directed by Jerry Cox, and many others. Each has tended to concentrate on a particular area of diagnosis and treatment. Probably the most complete single program is that of El Camino Hospital in California.

In 1966, El Camino Real Hospital, a 465-bed facility near Los Angeles, began to work with Lockheed Missile and Space Corporation to develop a total hospital information system. The system, which was later purchased by Technicon, has both hospital and patient management data, including such items as patient records, census, drug files, employee records, purchases, and all medical services including laboratory results. Hard copy is available at many locations. Areas covered by the program include the following:

| | |
|---|---|
| Nursing | Scheduling, availability of patient care plans |
| Admitting | On-line patient entry data |
| Radiology | Scheduling |
| | Access to charts via television |
| | Direct computer input x-ray data |

| Dietary | Diet order lists |
| Laboratory | Orders for laboratory tests of all results. direct input to computer |
| Records | Summarization and organization of medical records |
| ER | Registration of Emergency Records |
| Physician | Direct orders for patient on computer, patient records available immediately, use of problem-oriented records in treatment, improved accuracy of orders and diagnosis, immediate order transmittals, information and drug schedules, laboratory normal values, indication of therapy, billing, and insurance |

This total system permits control of all phases of hospital operation. The cost benefits are difficult to assign, but in general the use of the system has resulted in a savings of about $3 per bed per day. Despite the demonstrated effectiveness of the system, it was accepted at first by only 60 percent of the physicians but by up to 95 percent of the other hospital personnel.

The system has two devices to communicate with a central computer: (1) television screen, lightpen, and keyboard; and (2) multiprinter. The first device is used by all personnel from many units scattered over the hospital with a secret identification code for entry to the system provided to each user. The television screen displays requested information, such as drug lists. Items are selected for patient care or further information with the lightpen. The physician can call up lists of procedures, drugs, etc., to plan a complete treatment. The computer then sends documentation to the proper department. The keyboard is used for such items as patient's names, number, insurance, etc. The multiprinter prints out lists of all sorts, including care plans, drugs, medications due, laboratory results, radiology reports, etc. The computer generates lists for nursing stations specifying hours when drugs should be given, correct dosages, lists of daily orders, reminders for overdue work-ups, etc. The patient care plan includes diet and fluid balance orders, drugs, treatments, lab orders, and notes, such as language difficulties. The computer reviews and computes the bill on a daily basis and prepares a discharge summary when the patient leaves.

This is by far the most sophisticated patient care system in existence and illustrates clearly two points: (1) telecommunications can create a revolution in health care and (2) a revolution is not always easily accepted by people who are set in the ways of delivering care.

The sociology of the system is very interesting. When the system was first installed, the nurses and other personnel adopted it readily but physicians refused to use it to any great extent. It required about 5 years before the physicians were willing to trust the system and use it daily. One of the main savings is in management. The flow of paper has been reduced to a trickle. Another advantage has been the auxiliary programs. The computer alerts the physician to drug overdosages, to incompatible drugs, and to other problems with the patient. It permits the planning of a total care package including all elements of diagnosis, treatment, and care as a unit operation. This may well be the hospital system of the future. The Technicon Corporation has recently purchased the system and is marketing it throughout the country.

Clearly, the advantages of having a structured and accessible medical record data base are numerous. First is the ability rapidly to retrieve information concerning a patient from a number of separate places. Second, with growing concern for both quality control and cost control, the ability to review these record data in several different ways is of significant advantage. Patient records may be reviewed for adherence to medical criteria or for the over- or underutilization of services. In manual systems that are unstructured, it is almost impossible to perform these tasks accurately, and when performed at all, they are extraordinarily time-consuming and expensive. Attempts to develop computer-based automated medical records for the hospitalized patient have been unsuccessful because of the complexity of data involved and the timeliness required in the care of these often critically ill patients. However, ambulatory care has fewer constraints, and most medical care given in the U.S. today is provided on an ambulatory basis from individual doctors' offices, group practices, and outpatient departments of hospitals. It is in these ambulatory settings that the major successes in developing automated medical records have occurred. This has been especially true in prepaid group practices, where patients' illnesses tend more to the acute and self-limiting or slowly progressive and chronic, and the environment is more controlled.

The major block to completing the development from a summary report to a complete medical record has been the inability to structure physicians' notes. While it has been possible to use coding schemes for diagnoses or problems, it has been much more difficult to structure physicians' notes concerning historical information and physical findings. Nevertheless, there has been considerable success in the implementation of automated medical record systems in ambulatory settings.

## CONTROL OF TECHNOLOGY

In the discussion of the use of high tech to save lives, as with heart transplants, kidney transplants, etc., the criterion has been survival. However, as Radimtoola (1983) pointed out, there are many degrees of recovery following cardiac bypass surgery. Patients may return to an active life, patients may still suffer with degrees of angina and some patients may not have been materially helped. But, obviously, they all survived; therefore, some other criterion must be devised to measure the quality of survival. Hellinger (1983) suggested the development of a QALY (Quality Adjusted Life Years) in which the years of survival are adjusted by a factor which takes into account the quality of life. On this basis many individuals who have survived high technology procedures have a very poor QALY. Patients on dialysis, for example, are clearly not normal in quality of life and the number of suicides among them clearly demonstrates the poor quality of the life they lead. Patients who must exist for long periods on high doses of very toxic drugs are another example. If we equate the QALY with the cost of the procedure, another measure may be obtained for the value of any procedure and may raise questions as to whether the procedure should be attempted.

## Are Solutions Possible?

The relation between the hospital and the physician is a strangely reciprocal one. On the one hand, the hospital could not operate without a professional staff. The patient flow is dependent upon the physician to attract patients and refer them to the hospital in which that physician has privileges. Therefore, the physician has a considerable hold on the hospital. The doctor can, at least theoretically, remove referred patients to another hospital at any time.

On the other hand, the hospital has certain powers which it more or less abrogates. Lawsuits have determined that the hospital is responsible for negligence on the part of physicians if it had the knowledge to restrain their actions. The hospital has certain powers as a result to restrict the physician. Certain hospitals have barred physicians with high mortality figures from operating. The hospital can, at least in theory, remove privileges from a physician but this, in fact, seldom happens.

Control is exerted or ought to be exerted by several means. Utilization review should locate those physicians who have exceeded the norms in patient stays or treatment. Some hospitals publish lists of patient stays by disease and by doctor in an attempt to coerce compliance. Continuous education on the costs of drugs and tests can be conducted by the staff. Publication of lists of physicians who overuse drugs and tests have been attempted. Crile has suggested the publication of mortality figures from surgery. Hospitals should maintain records of infection, accidents, and other untoward events which compromise the patient and these should be available for patient inspection. The accuracy and efficiency of laboratory analyses could be available to everyone including the number of repeat tests. Physicians should be given a total cost breakdown of the hospital and the charges which are made to the patient. Patient bills should be sent to the physician. In essence, this boils down to a greater information flow which would make everyone aware of the costs and charges and the likelihood of a successful procedure.

If we consider the hospital as a business, all of these reports would cost money not only in the production of the reports but in the decreased usage of hospital facilities. The end results, however, might be a reduction in the number of beds and the purchase of expensive equipment, all of which would be to the advantage of the patient.

Solutions also rest with the physician directly. It is possible to argue the advantages of the increase in surgery in this country as compared to comparable nations on grounds of better medicine and better diagnosis, although the death rates belie this contention. It is more difficult to argue that the poor need less surgery that the wealthy but such appears to be the case. There is a clearcut difference between those who are affluent and those who are not, in almost double the number of surgical procedures performed per unit of population (Bombadier, 1977). It is by no means clear that the nonaffluent group has a death rate twice as high as the rest of the country, which implies that much surgery is unnecessary. Closer examination of the cause and effects of surgery is essential.

The stand-alone surgical unit can be a valuable part of the health care system. In Manitoba, with the advent of National Health Insurance, some 55 percent of all surgery is done on an outpatient basis. Some 25 procedures can be performed and it has been estimated that $15 billion could be saved per year in this country with such a system. The Canadians claim that outpatient surgery is better not only because of the short time and low expense involved but also because the number of cross-infections are markedly reduced (Robinson, 1980). The major problem seems to be that if operations are performed on an outpatient basis in the afternoon, the patient may not have time fully to recover from the anesthesia before being sent home in the care of relatives (Laurie, 1964).

The relationship of technology to the health care system is illustrated in Figure 1 (page 13). The figure demonstrates clearly that as technology demands increase and more becomes available it increases the cost of care, makes the cost available to fewer people, decreases the cost benefits, and decreases the number helped. The situation can be illustrated by the data on by-pass surgery or heart transplants. The technique requires elaborate technology carefully used and the cost is tremendous. As a result, only a few people will ever have the operation. The same amount of money (say $2 billion) would innoculate millions of children against crippling diseases, launch a prevention campaign which could save millions from future heart disease, or provide health care in areas which do not have it.

*Chapter 6*

# ETHICS OF LIVING AND DYING

Medical ethics has been brought to the fore by malpractice suits and by the rising issue of rights of individuals and of informed consent. Doctors have been living with an ethic of practice since the time of Hippocrates but the new technological advances which permit them to keep a person alive, to save lives which would otherwise have been lost, and attempt repair of tissues which could not be touched a few years ago, have raised questions which have yet to be answered. Medical ethicists have posed such questions as:

How much effort should be placed in heroic methods to save lives? Should a person with a liver transplant receive 20 pints of blood though still with small chance of survival, when blood is in short supply for accident victims and other more cost-beneficial procedures? How much information should be given to the patient? Should patients be told they are going to die? Should all risks be pointed out to a patient about to undergo a procedure? How many patients are told that the risks are about 1 percent that they are going to die if they have an operation?

Is informed consent always obtained? Do patients really know what they are being subjected to in an operation, the actual risks, the postoperative complications, the chance of benefit, and the costs?

Should a non-MD always follow the MD's advice? This is a routine problem in the Emergency Room, where rapid decisions must be made and patients deteriorate rapidly.

How much leeway should be given to paraprofessionals?

Are patient rights more important than the rights of society?

Do we have the right because of the one-doctor/one-patient relationship to expend 9 percent of the medical resources on 1 percent of the patients as we do with heart transplants, bypass surgery, and liver transplants?

Do the rights of society in terms of prevention of diseases, costs of care, and chances of benefit outweigh those of an individual patient?

How are scarce resources to be allocated? This has been discussed above but other aspects can be mentioned.

Should we accord kidney dialysis to a senile individual who can contribute nothing to society?

Is abortion a medical or legal question? Can a woman decide about the function of her own body as for a hysterectomy but not about pregnancy?

Where do we draw the line between the desire to save lives and the quality of the life which will be saved?

Is all technology good? Where should the line be drawn between too much effort to maintain life by artificial means and the desire to "pull the plug" on the part of patient or family?

We can raise still more general questions in the same area.

Are two standards of care ethical? We have two standards, one for those who can pay and one for those who cannot pay. The operation of "Medicaid mills" in which patients received poor care and short shrift have been well documented by DHHS. The situation is now spreading to other areas. Physicians are taking fewer and fewer Medicaid assignments and are decreasing their coverage of Medicare. The situation is so bad that the federal government has suggested that a rule be adopted which requires a physician to provide service regardless of reimbursement (NCHR, 1983).

Is it ethical for the patient to be exposed to less than satisfactory medicine? A survey by the JCAH revealed that only 56 percent of patients were satisfied with their doctor, and 46 percent with the hospital and only 60 percent with the amount of information they received.

Questions can also be raised about the use of drugs. Some 55,000 patients received emergency treatment last year for overdosage of Valium, a tranquilizer prescribed in enormous quantities.

Finally, we may ask if it is ethical to practice in an overcrowded field where the only way to make a reasonable income is to charge high prices. We have 99,357 internists, 98,667 surgeons, and 94,940 general physicians in the country. Is this the correct proportion? Should we have more surgeons than general practitioners?

## THE ETHICAL COST OF LIVING

With any intensive care unit, two problems arise. The first problem is medical and economic. Should survival be a function of expenditure of a large part of the health care dollar for a few individuals? Should individuals with severe defects requiring perhaps a lifetime of care at the public expense be given every possible procedure? With the development of resuscitation and respiratory and life support systems, we have placed a great deal of power in the hands of the physician to maintain life. In every case the cost is very great. On the other hand, the ethics of the situation must also be considered. What is the right to life and the right to die as a moral issue? Is it moral to sustain the life of an individual for years (as in the case of Quinlan) when the individual is totally incapacitated and incapable of response? Is it morally correct to sustain the life of a spina bifida child to subject it to a life of pain, disease, and repeated episodes of hospital care?

On the other hand, we can cite many examples of the improvement of technology, which has resulted in costs without benefit, either ethically or medically. Budetti (1981) has surveyed the neonatal intensive care units of the country. In 1980, 200,000 infants were treated in intensive care and about 50 percent died. The survivors had serious defects. Some 20 percent had serious abnormalities which could be life-threatening. The total cost was $1.5 billion. There is considerable question as to the number of infants which should be placed in intensive care. The rates vary from about 8.5 percent in New York to less than 3.5 percent in Ohio. Many of these children have medical problems in later life. Some 40 percent of them are in the hospital within the first year of life while only 8 percent of normal children are so admitted. Costs have been estimated at $100,000 over the life of the child who also has a shortened life span and more medical problems than normal children. The costs of infant intensive care depends largely upon the birth date. In very premature infants the costs may reach $40,000 with a very high rate of mortality, and questions can be raised as to the economics and morality of saving the life of such children.

The difficulties of the newborn have been under close scrutiny in the last few months as a result of reports from several sources indicating that the number of children born with defects has doubled within the last 10 to 15 years. Federal legislation passed in 1975 has mandated federal support for such individuals and may be very expensive. It is estimated that the number of children enrolled in such programs has increased 15 percent the last 10 years and the cost has risen by more than $1 billion. John Marshall of DHHS (personal communication) has suggested that the cause may be the life styles of mothers (smoking, etc.), the inheritance of genetic disease (diabetes) from mothers who would not have reproduced in previous generations and the survival of infants who would otherwise have died without high technology utilized to preserve life. The situation is likely to become worse in the future. The survival of the fittest may be an old Darwinian theory but it still applies. When we allow the weakest members of the society to survive and reproduce we decrease the gene strength of future generations.

As a final comment, more than one-half of all children's deaths under the age of ten are due to accidents and some 400,000 children per year have some major disability as a result of accidents. Why should we spend more on the treatment of birth defects in children with a short life span than we do on children who have passed the critical period but who are denied becoming useful members of society as a result of negligence (Heller, 1976)?

We have mentioned the right-to-life and the right-to-die but recently there has been introduced the concept of "wrongful life" by which a couple sued a physician and hospital for maintaining the life of a child who had serious medical defects and again in another case for not recommending an abortion when the physician knew the fetus had serious defects. The decision went against the physician in each case (*Medical World News*, Dec. 13, 1976, p. 49).

Breast cancer has also created a surgical problem. Thousands of breast cancers are removed each year by two methods, a radical or a partial breast removal. The patient is placed in the hospital and a major operative procedure is set up. The tumor is biopsied and if negative the patient is released; if positive, the breast is operated upon. Schachter (1981) found that the cost of the operation could be reduced almost 25 percent by outpatient biopsy. This is now done in only a few cases but the savings are apparent. In addition, Cole, Crile, and others have found that partial mastectomies are equally effective for removing the tumor, require only 4 days instead of 13 in the hospital and result in overall saving of about $185 million per year.

The United States has many times the highest rate of hysterectomies in the world. Most other countries do about one-half the number done in the U.S. In 1981 the rate was about 817 operations per 100,000 women. The average cost was about $2,900. It has been estimated (Karenbrot, 1981) that the savings on future illness caused by retention of the uterus run about $1.4 billion while the operation itself costs about $2.9 billion (Cole, 1976).

When an ulcer is suspected in an individual, the procedure of choice is often an upper GI tract endoscopy. The average cost is $250. Showstock (1981) claims that the procedure is of doubtful value, that no trials have ever been conducted to determine its effectiveness, and that all of the information can be collected by other less expensive means.

We have often gone through similar procedural methods which on examination proved to be ineffective. The Wagensteen freezing method of stomach treatment was widely used a few years ago with some 2,500 machines in hospitals. It was proven to be totally ineffective in a controlled clinical trial and was totally abandoned. It may be that endoscopy will follow the path to oblivion along with much of the demand for inhalation therapy.

Renal failure is a fatal disease. Before the advent of the dialysis technique, death was the inevitable consequence of the disease. When Scribner at the University of Washington invented the dialyzer, the extent of the need was unknown. The dialyzer was intended only as a short-term support mechanism until kidney transplants could be arranged or until the patient recovered from a short term disease brought on by toxins. The dialysis mechanism rapidly became the method of choice when it was discovered that there was no possibility of obtaining enough kidneys for transplantation. At the moment about 75,000 patients are being dialyzed, many unwisely. Renal dialysis has become big business. National Medical Care, one of the leaders in the field of for-profit dialysis, grew from a $7 million a year company making no profits to a $150 million a year company making a profit of close to $20 million last year. The growth is due entirely to the Medicare program and its support of End Stage Renal Disease treatment. The unit director, an MD, makes in the neighborhood of $400,000.

The center depends upon a relationship with local MDs who are expected to refer their patients to the centers. There has been criticism that doctors without relationships with NMC may not be able to refer patients to the centers (Kolata, 1980).

Several problems have arisen in connection with the centers. In fact, the HCFA is debating the placing of a ceiling on payments for dialysis, which would sharply limit the income. Secondly, the centers are thriving as moneymaking organizations in spite of repeated demonstrations that patients can be dialyzed at home for about 30 percent of the cost in centers. However, it is the practitioner who determines whether a patient can be dialyzed at home or in the center and it is often more convenient for the doctor to choose the center which is usually located close to a medical complex. NMC has lobbied strongly against bills in Congress which would require the use of home dialysis for 50 percent of all patients.

Another problem with major kidney dialysis centers is that they often dialyze persons who do not need the treatment. Senile elderly patients, dying patients, and others have been dialyzed at high cost and low benefit. Scribner's original plan at Washington selected patients on the basis of community need, stage of disease, and other criteria but at the present time almost anyone can be dialyzed for long periods of time. There is also a question of survival. Many patients develop psychotic symptoms and go downhill regardless of treatment. This again raises the question as to whether we are dialyzing too many patients because the centers are available and insurance will foot the bill.

We are faced with another but similar problem. Patricia Harris, former Secretary of DHHS, announced in 1980 that the agency was investigating the cost and benefit of heart transplants to determine whether such a procedure fell within the reasonable and necessary provision of medical care. If the plan is adopted and Medicare will pay for heart transplants, the cost may be as high as $3.5 billion per year. The basic question again is does a high technology expensive project, which benefits only a very few, divert funds from low tech, high benefit projects for large numbers of people being healed with immunizations or preventive measures of other kinds. Blue Cross of California has already paid for some 20 heart transplants, so the decision is imminent.

If Medicare decides eventually to pay for heart transplants, will it also pay for heart-lung, liver, and other similar transplant procedures? If so, the costs may rapidly get out of hand. A few billion for kidneys, a few billion for hearts, a few billion for livers, and the Social Security budget may indeed be bankrupt and vital services which are much less visible and costly will be neglected.

When the kidney transplant program began, the average age of the recipients was under forty and less than 20 percent were over fifty years of age. With the advent of centers and Medicare payment the average age is now well over fifty (Kolata, 1980). Will the same hold true for transplantation of other organs? Will a transplant reward a person who has no more to contribute, for a life well spent, or should it be reserved for those who provide a cost benefit to society?

The United States has many more patients on dialysis than any other country in the world for the same amount of renal disease. Other countries discourage elderly patients from dialysis because once patients are placed on dialysis they are difficult to remove. Kolata (1980) tells of a case of an elderly woman placed on dialysis when comatose. She lived unconcious for months because the doctors were afraid to remove her from the machine without her consent, which she could not give. There are patients with heart disease and disseminated cancer who are still being dialyzed.

If we have 50,000 kidney patients with their resultant problems what will the situation be when this figure is multiplied by other thousands of lung, liver, and heart patients? And we must bear in mind that the largest part of any cost is borne by the taxpayer. How many individuals can afford a $100,000 operation and the attendant costs for a heart transplant?

The responsibility again rests with the physician. There would be no patients on dialysis or in other forms of high tech treatment if they were not assigned by the physician to the treatment. Physicians need to be educated to the costs and how much of that cost they pay through their taxes.

These problems bring others to mind. There is one area in which the hospital, the family, and the physician find benefit. The retention of the elderly patient in the hospital is of advantage to all except the patient and the cost of the system. The hospitalization followed by nursing home care is an expensive way to care for the elderly. It has been estimated that 70 percent of Medicare costs are expended on 9 percent of the patients. About 22 percent of the elderly are hospitalized at some time during the latter part of their lives and many of the hospital days are unnecessary (Campion, 1983).

## THE ETHICAL COST OF DYING

The physician is faced with a series of problems with the dying patient. Often the physician's decisions are modified by the family, by the hospital, and by society. There are some patients who want desperately to live and the physician has to balance this wish against a hopeless medical situation and the enormous cost of life support systems which can easily reach $1,000 a day. On the other hand, there are equally desperate patients who wish to die or to "pull the plug" but who are not allowed to do so by the family or by legal constraints or by the physician's fear of lawsuit.

Such cases are straightforward in their obvious circumstances but there are many other problems which are equally vexing but less obvious.

Is it ethically moral to undertake a program which will kill some but benefit many? The converse of the question also occurs regularly in health care and has been posed: is it ethical or moral to spend large sums to help one person when the same funds could help many people? At the base of this question is productivity. The productivity is obviously higher in the latter instance and with proper controls could be very high. Suppose the funds for the high technology needed for a heart transplant were used to initiate a preventive program related to heart disease so that the end result would not only be a reduction in the cost of high technology but an actual cost reduction as measured by a decreased number of heart attack victims?

A hyberbaric chamber costs $3 million per year to operate to care for about 900 patients. Could that $3 million be better spent in other care? Malaria kills about 3 million persons per year in India. DDT reduced the deaths to about 200 per year. When the manufacture of DDT was banned because of toxic effects, the death rates rose. Is this moral?

The community itself must be informed in order to make health care decisions in terms of facilities and dollars which affect all of its citizens. Data must be available in order that priority decisions can be made, and made well. We, as consumers, have not made such choices well in the past. More money has been spent on tuberculosis affecting 90,000 people and on polio affecting a few thousand than on venereal disease with 1,000,000 cases per year, because such decisions were often made on the basis of too little information.

The present health care system is oriented toward the producers and their needs and desires. The hours of medical care delivery are directed toward the hours which physicians normally work; the operating room is scheduled to their convenience. The health care delivery system in Jacksonville, Florida found that changing clinic hours from day to night markedly improved consumer participation (McLaughlin, 1975). Consumers know little about the delivery system. They are usually unable to determine how to get into the system, whether they are getting adequate care after entering it, and whether the charges are fair. The consumer must be taught not only to use the system wisely, but not to abuse it through overuse. Only the educated consumer can change the system to prevention rather than treatment of a particular disease entity. The success of the campaign to eradicate polio is a case in point. An intensive campaign with immunization almost eliminated the disease. It is now returning in some force because of consumer apathy and failure to communicate.

The rise of technology has resulted in a proliferation of laws and regulations which have no real scientific base. One of the most prevalent is genetic screening for such diseases as PKU. If a mother has defective genes should she be prohibited from having another child? If a fetus is known to bear defective genes should an abortion be *required*? Heart disease is probably linked to some genetic properties. Should potential victims be screened and regulated in dietary intake or by other means? And finally, a topic we shall return to again: who should make the decisions? In many cases they are now being made as political decisions, often without valid medical input, and as the costs of regulation, testing, and treatment soar, productivity decreases.

## FRAUD

Honesty in science and medicine has always been a hallmark of the profession. Galen, in ancient Greece, pointed out the necessity of honesty and the Oath of Hippocrates points up the physician's need to respond honestly to the patient. Within the last few years a spate of dishonesty has been brought to the public's attention. It is not certain whether this represents a great increase in dishonesty or whether it represents a more open society. Medicaid frauds in which several physicians have been indicted for criminal offenses and the relatively large number of scientists who have been suspected of falsifying data may indicate

**Table 5    Examples of Fraud in Medical Practice in Several Locations**

| Location | Kind of Fraud |
|----------|---------------|
| California | Billing patient for unperformed services |
| Massachusetts | Bills of 1,800 Medicaid patients who did not exist |
| Maryland | Dentist charged with false billing |
| Illinois | Fraudulent Medicaid claims |
| New York | 175 pharmacists charged with false billing |
| Texas | Laetrile used for cancer treatment |
| Michigan | 6,000 laryngoscopies in two years |

a trend. All cases of fraud represent a loss of productivity. The cost of redoing the work is expensive, the cost of checking work by others requires time and effort, and the public may have lost in fees paid or unnecessary treatments. This problem is of particular interest when data are falsified in drug trials because the acceptance of a drug based on faulty data may endanger others for years to come (Table 5).

## THE JUDICIARY

The interference of the judiciary in the scientific process regardless of the motive has seriously impeded productivity in many cases. The problem is compounded by the fact that most government bureaus which ultimately may be sued are deliberately inflating risk factors in order to protect themselves and perhaps the public. The setting of a standard for x-ray exposure below that which the normal individual would accumulate from surrounding radiation in the course of a normal life is a case in point. It is not unusual to ban saccharine or other drugs because enormous doses in test animals reveal some hint of danger. It is common to set standards at one-tenth of the dosage which causes some detectable change. We need to revise federal laws on acceptable risks and we may someday want to ask for a decision on the basis of popular vote.

It should be remembered that avoiding risks is not riskless. OSHA has banned some procedures which the FDA considers essential for proper safety. When most substances are considered harmful until proven safe the associated costs may become unacceptable.

Another region in which the courts have entered without justification and with possible harm has been the area of withholding medical treatment (Kolota, 1979). In order to decide upon the merits of a particular case, the case must be tried in court and this ruling, in turn, becomes the precedent. Doctors have been afraid to issue orders not to resuscitate an incompetent or dying patient. There is a record of one woman being resuscitated 70 times in 24 hours before she finally died. The cost must have been enormous. We are now faced with the legal question of abortion and whether an ovum is a person at the time of fertilization. There is no question that the birth of damaged children results in heavy burdens on society for the long term. Should a woman be required to have an abortion if it can be shown that birth will result in such a burden? It is rare that a family can afford the expense of maintaining such an individual without public support of some sort. There is no doubt that ICUs operate in many cases to sustain the life of unsavable patients. Results suggest that 85 percent of very ill ICU patients die within a year. If this is true it must be apparent that heroic measures are being taken at great cost to maintain life. When 25 percent of total costs of a hospital may be invested in the ICU, a close examination of the admitted patients and a screening for possible recovery might be in order. Without a doubt, the doctor practices "defensive" medicine and a part of the problem is the legal system. (See malpractice below). One of the problems of defensive medicine on the part of the doctor and the hospital is the exorbitantly large awards made in the medical cases. It is not uncommon to have awards for millions of dollars which is far more compensation than should ever be considered. The usual excuse is that a large company has been at fault and should be made to pay. But if the hospital is forced to pay, the costs of medical care rise.

## MALPRACTICE

It has been established that malpractice costs the hospital system or the U.S. about $1 billion per year in insurance and that individual physicians such as the neurosurgeon may pay $10,000 or more in premiums. The cost is passed along to the patient. Here is one case in which the culprit can be easily spotted—the trial lawyer. While there is no doubt that many cases of malpractice do exist in the hospital and physician's office, it is claimed that 40 percent of all cases may be frivolous and without merit. The contingency fee has brought the lawyer into the field. Awards of millions of dollars provide a lucrative income for the malpractice bar. The facts are clearly demonstrated by the situation in Great Britain, where contingency fees are not allowed and where malpractice suits are 1 percent of those in this country and awards are even less. It is true that some real causes of malpractice may escape punishment in Great Britain because of this situation but it is more productive for the whole system.

Part of the malpractice problem is the doctor. The failure to explain procedures to the patient, the failure to follow standing orders, the refusal to keep up with the field all lead to a situation which condones malpractice. The most common fault is the assumption that a medical certification may qualify a physician for any medical procedure regardless of the fact that the certification may have been issued 40 years ago and techniques changed radically since that time.

Medical malpractice occurs for several reasons. Technical errors due to poor technique may be one source. Judgmental errors which arise because of poor strategy in handling cases are another source of malpractice. Normative errors where the responsible party has taken an imprudent action which does not conform to the norms of society or the profession constitutes still another form of error. Finally, error may arise from exogenous sources where the patient may not have followed orders or where something happened which was beyond the control of the system.

There has been one major advantage to the malpractice issue, and one of less advantage. The major advantage is that surgery has been reduced some 25 percent by physicians who probably should not be performing surgery in the first place and the secondary advantage is the greater care taken in handling cases even though much of this care is "defensive" and may be unnecessary. The disadvantage is that defensive medicine may mean additional procedures which are dangerous or unnecessary and thus decrease productivity.

Lombardi (1978) has suggested that the number of malpractice suits is related to the number of law graduates and, in fact, if a plot is made of increases in claims versus the number of graduates, there is a direct relationship. This is a serious matter since it has been estimated that $7 billion is spent for defensive medicine over and above that necessary for good medical care. The Commission on Medical Malpractice has reported that 45 percent of all suits received some payment and of the 45 percent which were paid, the insurance companies believe that 40 percent were actually meritorious and deserved payment. The insurance companies also reported that of about 2,500 successive cases, 1,596 were overcompensated for injury and 477 were undercompensated. That raises real questions about the quality of suits and the action of courts and awards for injuries. The situation is further complicated by the distribution of malpractice cases. Most cases, and those carrying the biggest awards, occur in California and New York. A few hospitals and physicians account for most of the cases and 87 percent of all physicians and hospitals have never been sued. Evidence by DHHS and other agencies suggest that malpractice may be *underestimated*. Five percent of all physicians are said to be dishonest or incompetent and 1.5 percent are addicted to some drug. These lower quality physicians see about 12 million patients a year and it would be surprising if there are not many unrevealed cases of malpractice.

Although we usually assume that the physician is to blame in cases of malpractice, actually about 75 percent of all malpractice cases originate in hospitals and 88 percent of all payments are for injuries incurred in hospitals. Twenty-nine percent of cases are due directly to hospital negligence. However, if the physician is at fault within the hospital, the hospital can control the MD only through admitting procedures, and often hesitates to take this step because it limits patient flow. Hospitals should have the responsibility to monitor quality in the unit and should exert tightened control.

Many solutions have been suggested to remedy the malpractice situation. Several states have adopted forced arbitration as a means of reaching a fast equitable decision. Other states have proposed no-fault insurance, but this has not been very successful because many states limit no-fault recovery to about $35,000 in such cases and this is often insufficient for medical expenses.

A major problem with the threat of malpractice is that the physician feels forced to alter the method of treatment (Tancredi, 1978). Data indicate that the average doctor considers malpractice in more than 70 percent of patients seen and alters treatment accordingly. A survey of practicing physicians in 1975 by *Medical Economics* found that out of fear of malpractice, physicians ordered more tests than they thought necessary, asked for consultations when in the slightest doubt, hospitalized more patients than normally, and more importantly, did not accept the "high risk" patient, thus placing a part of the population in jeopardy to protect self-interest.

## ETHICS OF THE HEALTH CARE SYSTEM

In a very real sense the ethics of the system of health care are rooted firmly in money and the prospect of profit. It must be remembered that a "nonprofit" hospital actually makes about a 10 percent return on investment per year. If it did not it would be unable to buy expensive equipment, build new wings, pay off existing debt, etc. Every administration keeps an eye on the bottom line. As a result, several practices can be listed which are obviously not to the benefit of the patient but which are routine practice in hospitals (Kinzer, 1980).

The system is designed to have the biggest return for those who do the most for the patient. Individual piecework charges for hospital service automatically increase the costs.

Hospitals believe with some justification that spending more money for additional equipment results in more intake of funds and this again raises costs at both ends.

Hospitals actually started Blue Cross in order to create a group of patients who didn't care about the price and therefore had no compunction about high charges.

Hospitals encourage the use of services to the limit available. An empty bed is a costly bed, and unused CAT scanners cost more than $1,000 a day. Services which are available must be used.

Supply of medical services is open-ended. We can always supply any additional demand by increasing resources.

The hospital has no effective control on orders by physicians or on physicians' demands for equipment or services.

The hospital does not relate incomes or outcomes of treatment to the price charged for a given service.

It should be apparent that a truly ethical system would examine the need as determined. The fact that this does not happen is in a sense unethical.

Finally, we must remember that the hospital supplies the services but that the physician orders them and has ultimate responsibility.

## ETHICS AND THE PATIENT

The practice of medicine until the 1970s was essentially strictly professional. The physician decided what was right for the patient, dictated the treatment, and the patient was assumed to accept the treatment without argument and to pay the bill without recourse.

With the wakening of consumer interest through Ralph Nader and others in the early 1970s the situation changed drastically. The patient became part of the system and demanded rights which had previously been denied without a thought. The medical record is a case in point. The medical record has been sacrosanct for hundreds of years. No patient was allowed to see the record and it was assumed to be the property of the hospital or physician. A series of court decisions changed the picture. The record was declared to be a part of the patient and to belong to the patient personally. The patient has a right to inspect the record, to take it from place to place, and to raise questions about its contents. Secondly, the patient became part of the procedure known as "informed consent." As a result of failure of disclosure before radical surgery, experimental treatment of patients without their knowledge, and similar practices, laws were passed which forced the professional to tell the patient of the procedures to be accomplished, the possible dangers, and the expected results.

Many difficulties resulted. Some physicians resented the need to secure the patient's consent and essentially refused to comply with the law. Others obeyed the law by breach rather than by observance. The complication of providing consent forms in readable English or in the language of the patient was a major problem. Hospitals always had consent forms but they were essentially a license to open treatment since no details were provided, and the signer gave the physician the right to initiate any treatment in the patient's best interest as determined by the physician.

On another level, the patient is querying medical decisions. The "right to life" and the "right to die" issues are often in direct conflict with the codes of the medical profession and have created considerable turmoil. The request of families to "pull the plug" on relatives considered incurable has strained relations within the system.

We have mentioned the right to a second opinion and although few individuals actually seek such an opinion at the present time, the trend seems to be to increase the number in that unions and some insurance companies are now requiring a second opinion before paying bills.

Many systems are now resorting to committees to make some of these patient-physician ethical decisions. They are not totally satisfactory because each person comes to the board with individual biases (Brown, 1980).

There are many medical decisions which affect society as a whole and which are deeply imbedded in ethics. The rebellion against vasectomy in India and contraception in South America are cases in point. The present battle over abortion and the conditions under which it should be performed has become more a political than a medical problem. The same sort of problem faces society when the question is raised about whether society should support treatment for lung cancer which the individual has brought upon him or herself by smoking, cirrhosis of the liver through alcoholism, or heart disease through obesity. Should medicine adopt procedures which are desired by society, but which may in the end damage the patient? Laetrile is the best example. A great deal of research has been performed to prove the compound worthless at a considerable cost to the taxpayer.

Some indication of the problem which IRBs (Institutional Review Board) face in dealing with patient use on research projects is suggested by the fact that only 21 percent of forms from hospitals were complete, and the procedures to be performed were not mentioned in 30 percent of the cases. In fact, more than 70 percent of all consent forms implied or stated that the risk was minimal. Less than 50 percent of the forms offered to answer questions (Gray, 1978). These data suggest that we have not yet been fully ethical in explaining to patients the treatment which they must undergo.

## ETHICS AND HEALTH CARE

Care of the patient varies widely from area to area. Some 15 percent of the hospitals in the country have about 50 percent of all claims for malpractice and it has been said that 75 percent of all patients incur some damage in those hospitals. Laws do not have the "teeth" to close such locations. Physicians are to blame. It has been estimated that a heart surgery unit which does not do several operations per month has a mortality rate which is three times that of another unit which performs more operations, yet this does not prevent the continued operation of the former unit. There is no way in which the patient can be informed of "bad" doctors. The medical profession protects its own and the number of doctors disqualified averages about 100 or so per year in a profession with 350,000 members. Every doctor knows of cases of malpractice by physicians who are shielded by their colleagues from disclosure.

A major problem in dealing with right to live or right to die cases is the failure of the courts to be consistent. The decisions have varied over a wide range.

Massachusetts has issued decisions which imply that a doctor must ask the court for permission before withholding treatment from an incompetent person. There appears to be little question but that competent persons can refuse medical treatment if they wish. Certain lawyers have argued that the courts are fairer and more objective than physicians or family in making such decisions and should be required to make them. This, of course, takes the practice of medicine from the doctor and places it in the hands of the court. A major risk for the doctor comes about because the majority of patients who are competent always opt for treatment and therefore it may be unethical to decide that an incompetent patient should not have treatment.

There are other less clear cases. It has been reliably estimated that a premature infant weighing less than 1,800 grams will cost the state or society more than $100,000 during the rest of its life because of incurable medical problems. In addition, the costs of sustaining life in such a patient are very great—up to $50,000. Should the physicians make the heroic efforts which are often undertaken to save such children (Boyle, 1983)? The ethical position is clear. Should a physician perform a procedure of doubtful efficacy on any patient? Should treatment be restricted in nonexperimental situations to known methods of proven worth? The second opinion may be the best treatment of choice in most major surgery. There are other elements to consider.

The present suits brought by the Federal government on behalf of "Baby Doe", requiring the doctor to do everything possible for severely handicapped newborns with resulting high costs and high continual upkeep on such patients for the foreseeable future, are another example of interference of government and the legal system in the practice of medicine.

We are rapidly losing our trust in the physician. Treatment is in the final analysis a placing of life into the hands of the doctor and many consumers are now having second thoughts about its desirability without second opinions, further consultations, or severe questioning. Patients are also questioning the financial relationships. In earlier days, it was assumed that the physician knew best and made the wisest and cheapest selection of care. That is not now the case. Specifically, questions are being raised about several hundred-thousand-dollar incomes among physicians and the charges which must be assessed to reach that income level.

One of the major problems confronting the physician is the rapid proliferation of toxic materials. California has listed some 800 chemicals which are considered highly toxic and there are undoubtedly several thousand more. Most doctors are not trained in medical school in the field of toxicology and as a result they pay little attention to the environmental factors which may ultimately prove to be more important than medical factors in the treatment and cure of disease. Is the physician ethically bound to learn about those problems and their impact on medical treatment?

*Chapter 7*

# THE PHYSICIAN AND THE HEALTH CARE SYSTEM

Physicians do not usually consider any part of the health care system beyond their own offices and the hospital. The tremendous expansion of nursing homes has occurred with little attention from the medical profession. Only 36 percent of homes have regular physician visits and only 54 percent have physicians on call. The average physician spends less than 66 minutes a month in nursing homes (Solan, 1974). In 1981 the Federal government paid about $24 billion for nursing home care and about $500 million for home help. The services were used by about 2.4 million people.

In Great Britain the nursing home as such does not exist. However, the population uses a great deal of home care. The visiting nurse and the physicians treat patients at home for conditions which would merit hospital stay in the United States. Home health care is not used to any extent in the U.S. but is increasing slightly.

The proper combination of home help and nursing homes could materially reduce the costs of care. Pre-admission review of patients could reduce costs in nursing homes by as much as 20 percent (Knowlton, 1982) and home care could reduce the nursing home costs by about 35 percent. Finally, the use of the hospice rather than the hospital for the dying patient could materially reduce cost, because about 80 percent of the deaths of elderly occur in the hospital (Cohen, 1979; Maloney, 1983). Garrell (1983) has proposed that we educate the physician to care of the geriatric patient by establishing geriatric residencies which would both improve medical care in general for the elderly and improve care in nursing homes where the residencies would be conducted. This may be a critical issue in the future as the number of elderly increase, and doctors must become aware of the problem. Carels (1980) estimated that 80 percent of all physicians have no idea of the use of such ancillary care for their patients.

## THE PHYSICIAN, THE PATIENT, AND HEALTH CARE

We have placed a great deal of blame for rising and uncontained costs in the health care system upon the physician. However, the patient must accept a considerable part of the blame and is in many ways abetted by the physician in the failure to contain costs.

The evidence is clear that the physician issues prescriptions but the patient fails to take them. Less than 50 percent of prescriptions are filled and still fewer are taken by the patient after the doctor issues the order. There are several reasons for this. One, of course, is the high cost of drugs. Secondly, a major reason is the lack of information. Too often the prescription is issued with only a cursory explanation of the need, the side effects, and the expected results. There is little incentive for the patient to take the drug.

The patient has high expectations of the health care system (McGee, 1981). The TV and related information sources daily report the miracles of medicine and encourage the patient to believe in the magic cure. The public is rarely told about the poor results which may ensue or about the costs of the procedure. As a result, the patient usually demands "the best" even when the physician sees no real point to recommending a particular procedure. Patients demand to be kept in the hospital, to have body scans, and perhaps surgery, and the physician practicing defensive medicine is afraid to refuse because exacerbation of the problem without all possible recourse could result in a suit for malpractice.

Again, patients are unwilling to take care of themselves or their families. In most of the countries of the world other than the United States the elderly and the bedridden are taken care of at home with necessary visits from nurses and physicians. America has developed the nursing home concept to avoid the high cost of the hospital for chronic conditions but at the same time to avoid caring for the patient at home. The best example is in kidney dialysis. Virtually all of the kidney dialysis in the country is performed in renal dialysis centers. These centers cost about $35,000 per patient per year. Home dialysis is actually more convenient, perhaps safer and more psychologically beneficial at a cost of about $8,000 per year (Wauter, 1983). However, only 8 percent of all renal patients are being dialyzed at home. There have been complaints about inconvenience, need for training, and other excuses. None of them are valid.

Patients have no problem with accepting the high cost solution to their problem. It has been remarked that a large part of the bill is paid by insurance of one sort or another (Anderson, 1975; Dicker, 1983). As long as the bills are not presented, the patient is unconcerned about the costs. It has been clearly demonstrated, many times, that if co-insurance is introduced, the demand for services decreases with the increase in co-insurance charges. It has been argued that co-insurance is unfair in that it places an added burden upon those who cannot afford to pay, but at the same time we must remember that few patients can afford $35,000 for a kidney dialysis, $100,000 for a transplant, $2,500 for a pacemaker, etc., so that the higher cost technologies are paid for by taxation and insurance charges regardless of the economic status of the patient. It might be possible to return to the original days of the renal dialysis development at the University of Washington and choose by committee those who should have the service without copayment or to determine the amount of copayment to be collected from each patient.

Finally, the patient attempts to second-guess the physician. The evidence is clear that patients learn about most medical advances from TV and that they believe much of what they hear.

It has been estimated that the public gets 40 percent of its information about drugs from the media and that 60 percent of all drug advertising is misleading and may be dangerous. The over-the-counter (OTC) market runs into the billions as patients try to dose themselves, and more potent drugs (e.g., cortisol) are being placed on the market without a prescription.

The physician could act to alleviate most of the described problems. A major missing element in the health care system is information, and when physicians spend an average of 10 minutes with each patient they are unable to provide such.

It has been suggested that as the supply of physicians expands and competition becomes stronger we may see a change in the attitude of the physician (Smith, 1972). Although the pressure of numbers is unlikely to reduce costs in the near future for reasons already discussed, it is likely that the physician will have to compete in terms of better patient rapport, better service, more information, and more contact with the patient. A contravening force in the form of PPOs and HMOs will reduce prices by the kind of service that will force the patient into a mold of requiring use of a specified group of physicians.

Berkonovic (1976) listed the problem between physician and patients. The major complaints are still with us but increasing numbers of physicians may lead to some alleviation of the situation. Berkonovic listed:

Difficulty in obtaining appointments

Problems in seeing a doctor without an appointment

Length of time required to obtain an appointment and to see the doctor

Rude treatment from doctor and staff

Failure of the doctor to provide adequate information

Generally poor doctor-patient relations

## PHYSICIAN SUBSTITUTES AND THE PATIENT

There are other means of lowering the cost of health care. The substitution of PA and NP for physicians can make a major difference in health care delivery. Doerman (1975) and Falter

(1976) have pointed out the advantages of using NPs in rural areas and in other locations. When questioned, hospital administrators thought that NPs would be an advantage in their hospitals and would lower costs, but less than 40 percent admitted that they would even consider hiring an NP. Physician pressure on the hospital and through county medical societies effectively prevents the use of the NP except in a few states. One of the reasons is the problem of legal status. The NP who acts under the jurisdiction of a physician may make the doctor liable for malpractice in the event of a poor decision. The question of payment also arises. Should a NP doing the same job as a physician be paid the same? This has not been the case in the past and reports of the use of NPs suggest that savings of up to 40 percent can be achieved with no apparent decrease in quality of care, with NPs rendering a large part of the total care in remote areas.

LeRoy (1981) reported on the effectiveness of nurse practitioners in office practice. There are about 18,000 physician extenders in various categories. In general these are of two types. One type is certified by examination or board review and the second usually has a Master's degree in nursing. The nurse practitioner in particular has provided both a substitutive and complementary function. They are capable of providing a high percentage of primary services with proficiency equal to the physician's. The element which is usually in dispute is productivity. The NP can obviously deliver health care and increase productivity but may well not be utilized to the fullest extent. However, in some situations it has been estimated that the NP could save about $1 billion in health costs under proper conditions. NPs do spend longer with patients and see fewer patients in a given time, but, on the other hand, they also provide greater counselling service and better health education than the physician. All of the current data suggest the advantages of using the NP in office practice. Despite the available information, it is likely that the increase in the number of NPs will be small and that the number of physicians will increase at a much faster rate. This, in turn, is likely to restrict use of NPs as physicians need to find work as their numbers increase above those needed in the country.

Although Abdellah (1983) and others have pointed out the role to be played by the nurse practitioner and the physician's assistant, problems still arise. The most common difficulties listed include:

> A poor definition of the responsibility of the NP or PA in the system
>
> Poor supervision by the physician both in terms of too little or too much supervision
>
> Excessive work loads imposed by physicians
>
> The failure to develop good protocol for handling patients with or without physician supervision
>
> The failure to keep good records
>
> The tendency to spend more time with the patient than many physicians think warranted

As a result, several programs have not been a success and have closed. In other locations, many states have prohibited the hiring of the NP or PA except directly by the physician. When these objections to PA or NP performance are coupled with the oversupply of physicians, there is little wonder that the doctor is less than enthusiastic about the profession.

The relationship of the hospital, the physician, and the physician's assistant is political in nature. The physician is always confronted by politics. In solo practice the doctor is faced with competition from colleagues, and in a group practice starts out as the low man on the totem pole. In the hospital, doctors may be in conflict with the administrator about standards of care. They must deal with the vagaries of Congress in the reimbursements for Medicare and Medicaid patients. They must provide the best available care within the constraints of hospital pressure, peer pressure, and patient pressure. It is not an easy task. There is little wonder that they resent intrusions by additional health care professionals.

*Chapter 8*

# CONTROL OF THE HEALTH CARE SYSTEM

Nonprofit organizations suffer from several major problems which hinder efficient operation and lead to abuse of the tax-payers' funds. Most large nonprofit organizations find it difficult to establish objectives. In nonprofit organizations there is no overall direction from the top down and the lower echelons have different objectives and different ways of approaching the organizational objectives from those in top management. As a result, a certain degree of chaos always exists. One of the major problems which cannot be too often mentioned is the failure of the nonprofit organization to establish concrete objectives. Such objectives *can* be established, and should be, if the organization is to accomplish any sort of movement. In addition, the tie between planning and implementation in nonprofit organizations is often so loose that the members of the organizations cannot see results and cannot determine if anything they do makes a real difference.

Another major problem is the measurement of benefits in nonprofit organizations (Griffith et al., 1973). Most nonprofit organizations measure structure or function but do not consider outcomes (Fig.6). It is true that outcomes are often hard to de-

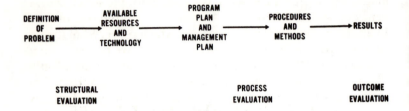

**Figure 6.**   **The process of evaluation pointing up the development of structural, process, and outcome evaluation and the successive improvement in evaluation with better methods.**

termine and to assign to any definite effort on the part of the organization. In health care, this should be a simpler matter than it has appeared to be. Health objectives should be easily stated and evaluated but it is easier to outline the number of cases treated, or the number of beds filled rather than to evaluate whether those cases have benefited.

It is often difficult to determine the extent to which an outcome is attributable to medical care. Many factors influence health and well-being: age, sex, race, geographic location, occupation, education, income, nutrition, and housing. Because of these complex interrelationships, we do not know how to measure a desired result in a particular situation. Many years may elapse before the effect of management on a certain disease becomes evident and by then new and different factors enter the situation.

Any discussion of organization and management in health care must be based on the realities of the system as it exists.

As a first approximation the system is designed to be infinitely expandable. As better care and new techniques are developed, the system expands to accomodate them. As users demand greater and greater levels of care and greater costs, the system again expands. We have never reached the point where the system has balked at greater expense or greater service even when it has been clearly demonstrated that greater costs do not necessarily mean better quality of service.

Secondly, all incentives are oriented toward higher cost care.

The physician demands the new technology, the hospital administrator must compete with the rival down the street, the patient demands the best care. All tend to raise the cost of care. In addition, the insurance companies which collect from the patient and pay the hospital or the physician have no incentive to reduce costs. The financing is open-ended and therefore costly.

Thirdly, the production units are poorly organized. The physician is for all practical purposes a small independent businessperson engaged in a limited production enterprise. The doctor is not in competition with anyone (who has seen a physician advertise "Appendectomies for $49.95 this weekend"?) Imposed upon this private business is the user who has no standard of quality except costs. The patient has no basis of comparison between hospitals or doctors and cannot make a value-judgment. There is no monitor on the outcomes of treatment so the patient has no feedback to determine the quality of the product received.

Fourthly, the service rendered depends upon the *system*, not on the user. The user of medical care has no criteria of judgment; therefore, the system sets the criteria. The consumer has no way to judge whether care could be provided at lower costs and, in fact, is usually told that low costs mean poorer care. Medical care is high style care and like high style fashions, the charges are greater. Like high fashion, the style changes from year to year.

Fifthly, as the cost of medical care increases, the cost of catastrophic illness increases more than the average. It has been estimated that 1 percent of the population uses 25 percent of the resources, largely because of the high technology of the ICU and similar high cost hospital services. Like any business, the system of health care behaves as it does because it is rewarded for such behavior by increased income, increased patient loads, and higher prestige.

## Costs and Benefits

Health care is funded by two means. In the first case, the funding occurs within a definite budget restriction, and in the second case, there is no budget set for the project. Examples would be funds allocated to the National Cancer Institute in the first case and the Medicaid budget in the second case. In the case of a fixed budget, trade-offs must often be made on the basis of cost effectiveness. Although such restrictions do not appear to apply to the second case, they apply indirectly because continual increases in open-ended budgets eventually force restrictions on the part of Congress or create protests from the taxed public (Fig. 7).

Two other questions may be raised about the determination of cost benefit. We may consider cost-benefit which is the true benefit resulting from the expenditure of funds, or we may consider cost effectiveness which is the determination of whether an expenditure of funds produces an effective result. The two are mutually inclusive but not totally overlapping. We may be concerned about the benefit of spending $500,000 per case to treat a given disease but that has nothing to do with the effec-

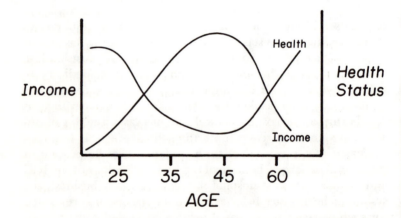

Figure 7.   The relationship between health, income, and age. Health is scaled from good at the bottom to poor at the top and income from low to high, illustrating that the period of health care need is also the period of lowest income (taken from Brown, *Politics of Health Care*, Cambridge: Ballinger Press, with permission).

tiveness of the treatment. On the other hand, we may raise questions about whether two procedures which cost the same are equally effective in outcomes.

In health care we must also take into consideration other aspects of the problem of cost. An attempt to affect the cost of a system and the benefit arising from the expenditure of funds can be approached from either the supply or the demand side of the economic problem. We can reduce the cost of hospital care by reducing the number of beds available, thus reducing the daily cost of supply, or we can induce the consumer or the physician to use fewer beds or to use them more wisely, thus reducing demand.

Although the medical system in the past years has been concerned largely with supply rather than demand, the rising cost of health care is gradually forcing attention to the question of demand and the limitation of demands.

Control of the system must occur in a finite time frame. This suggests that control can occur before the fact—preliminary control; during the operation—concurrent control; and after the fact—retrospective control. There are many examples of each in the health care system. Preliminary control occurs before the fact. The hospital may determine the number of operating rooms in use, the level of fire protection, dietary control, and the results to be expected in the laboratory. Concurrent control permits a constant check on ongoing procedures. The use of blanks in the hospital laboratory along with standards permits a constant ongoing control of procedures. The attendance of nurse and their duties are under concurrent control as are the changes in staffing, food supply, etc., to meet the daily census of patients. In business, retrospective control is not greatly emphasized but it is the most important control exerted in the health care industry. The regulations laid down by the federal government and other agencies and review bodies all constitute retrospective control. Determination as to whether the regulations were met can be made only after the procedure is completed. The basic objective of the PRO (Professional Standard Review Organization) is to review individual cases after physicians have performed their task to see if the work meets the standards of the medical community. On the other hand, the process of utilization review (UR) uses all forms of control. The length of stay in a hospital is set beforehand by the physicians as a group, the admission of the patient is reviewed on entry for length of stay, and the review takes place again at a later date to see if the desired stay was obtained. Preliminary control is set by the issuance of standards and regulations. The control process consists of a regular series of steps. The environment changes and, as a result, some change in performance occurs. A disparity occurs between the performance and the norms set by the organization and this places a strain in the operational structure. As a result, the organization changes to respond to the environment. The change made returns the system to normal or it may set in motion a new set of environmental alterations and a repetition of the cycle.

There is little point in controlling a situation or process unless evaluation is used to determine whether standards were actually met and when the process fell short of the desired goal. In the health care field, we have not looked closely at the process of evaluation. A part of the reason is that there is no overall health policy to which results can be compared.

Evaluation of a system comprising men and machines always consists of some combination of factors of structural evaluation, process evaluation, and outcome evaluation. True evaluation requires comparison of at least two systems: the existing system with a previous system or with a theoretical ideal. Even when such comparisons are valid, evaluation of health system outcomes are most difficult. Comparability of systems is always in question. Measurement of outcomes in health are difficult because morbidity or even mortality as an outcome is hard to define and hard to measure because criteria are often in doubt. Outcomes are strongly affected by factors other than the system under test, and often give no clue as to which elements of the system are producing the observed differences.

Because of these difficulties, evaluations are often based on process variables. These are measurable characteristics which effect the outcome in a predictable way. For example, reducing the time between notification of an emergency and arrival at the hospital can be expected to reduce morbidity and mortality. A process evaluation may not measure the degree of improvement of outcome due to the improvement in process. When the Jacksonville EMS was established, the number of persons surviving myocardial infarction dramatically increased during the transportation phase and 38 percent more died in the hospital. The process measurement indicated a marked improvement in transportation while an outcome evaluation would appear to be much less successful.

## THE ZERO SUM GAME

The provision of health care is a zero sum game if we assume that health care represents a fixed 10 percent of the GNP; if one portion of society spends more on health care, some other must spend less. We now spend about 25 percent of the health care dollars on the 5 percent of the population in intensive care. The zero sum means that we must spend less on the high technology to improve the chances of survival and better diagnosis of the last 1 percent of all cases and spend more on better care for all of the population. A city which has seven CAT scanners for a population of 1 million when one per 1 million population is sufficient is playing the zero sum game in the wrong direction. Unfortunately, jealous boards, politics, and pride are likely to obstruct changes in the system (Thurow, 1980).

Dual control affects the nonprofit organization. This is particularly true in the hospital where the two lines of command (the administrator and the chief of the medical staff) are often at odds over purchase of equipment, services rendered, or cost projections. The quality of control extends outside the organizations. A hospital has responsibility to its clients—the patients—and also to the board of directors and perhaps the community as a whole. Such dual responsibility leads to confusion. It may be apparent to the medical community and the government that a new CAT (Computerized Axial Tomograph) scanner is the last piece of equipment to be added to the armamentarium but if the hospital across the street has one, the board and the staff will insist on competing on the same level of services. The attempt on the part of an administrator to close an inefficient maternity service in favor of the one across the street may lead to confrontation by mothers-to-be and the staff.

Because of these conflicting aims and desires, the hospital and the health care system tend to focus on inputs in terms of patients or on outputs in terms of number of patients rather than on the true criteria of whether a health care system really works. In addition, the system is plagued by enormous control systems which often hamper rather than improve the overall efficiency. Regulations are imposed by accrediting agencies, by the city, the state, and the federal government, each of which may have established regulations in conflict with the other. The system is further confronted by changes in the political and social environment which may drastically alter circumstances.

Government regulations are blamed for many evils in the health care system and, in fact, may be responsible for some of them but every evil has a corresponding good. Workers want regulation on cost of care but oppose regulations on wages. Administrators want exactly the opposite. But all economy is regulated. The basic question is how much is too much. We complain about OSHA regulations as unreasonable, but no one wants 10,000 pages of documentation to make OSHA regulations work in every situation. A regulation which is fine in one context may be impossible in another.

The major regulation in health care has been the attempt to fix prices and costs (Krause, 1975). When prices are fixed, a zero sum game results as people benefit from the fixed prices, but the wages in the price fixed system cannot rise and some workers lose. If physician prices become too high, others may enter the competition (NPs, PAs, etc.) and regulations may be adopted to restrict development of these areas.

*Chapter 9*

# THE PHYSICIAN AND THE PATIENT

The old picture of the kindly, benign physician sitting beside the sick patient, making house-calls at night and serving as the family counselor has largely disappeared in favor of the business person who sees patients rapidly, is not well acquainted with them, and appears to have little regard for medical problems other than those related to the doctor's own specialty. Repeated interviews with patients reveal this picture, real or imagined, of the medical profession. Some investigators feel that family practice is growing largely because of the need of the patient to have closer contact with a specific physician or group. The development of HMOs also have some of this component phased on to the desire for lower costs of medical care.

The obligation of doctors to their patients breaks sharply into two major areas of controversy. On the one hand is a group of ethicists, physicians, and sociologists who believe that doctors have a moral obligation to serve the public including the poor. This group believes that since the practice of medicine is a monopoly conferred by licensing and training, the monopoly must provide for those who need service regardless of ability to pay. The future may bring a situation of oversupply of physicians, these critics say, and competition will increase, forcing aggressive patient-seeking on the part of the physician and the service rendered today may be returned in good measure later through good will generated. Sociologists claim that patients "expect" to receive care when they think they are ill and the physician should provide such care.

The second group believes that the physician is a worker in an industry and should be compensated for work performed as is the plumber or the lawyer. This group believes that the majority of patient ills are trivial or imaginary and a patient who wishes to see the doctor about such a condition should be prepared to pay for it.

It is likely that the truth lies somewhere in between. No physician should be asked to provide services at personal cost for trivial problems. Obviously, no doctor would refuse urgent care regardless of payment so the questions are raised about the borderline situations.

The situation is complicated by the economics of the system. Those who most need help are the least able to pay (Fig. 7, page 148). The provision of Medicare and Medicaid was structured for this group but the question is still not clear as to the extent of co-payment which should be expected or the physician's responsibility to provide low cost service.


## THE PATIENT AS A PERSON

The usual complaint of most patients is that the doctor does not provide enough information. This is probably due to two reasons: in the first place, many physicians consider themselves omnipotent and hesitate to reveal medical mysteries to their patients; and in the second place, the physician often does not realize how little information is conveyed by brief descriptions of illness in medical terminology. This lack of information carries over into the problem of "informed consent." The law requires and medical prudence dictates that a physician should inform the patient not only of the procedures to be done but also of the actual risks to be encountered in the treatment. All too often the latter point is neglected or omitted. This is particularly crucial in surgery where the patient is not informed of the mortality figures for an operation or the risk of postoperative complications.

The physician also neglects or deliberately avoids the situation of informing dying patients of their condition. There are two schools of thought on the problem. One suggests that the patient should be told and be allowed to prepare, the other holds that, in many cases, the patient should not be told.

The physician is confronted with the dilemma of the right to live or the right to die in many situations. In the elderly the decision to "pull the plug" is often not easy but in many cases can be left to the decision of the elderly patient. In children the decision becomes much more difficult. The cases in which religious beliefs have conflicted with the need for medical care have been decided both ways in the courts and there is no perfect answer. The decision to take heroic measures to sustain the life of a patient in the emergency room or the ICU may be in part a financial decision, which we have already discussed. Abortion presents a special case since both the political influences and the religious overtones have been brought to bear on a medical decision. Again decisions have gone both ways. Physicians have been sued for performing an abortion and they have been sued for *not* performing an abortion when a known medical defect existed. The age of consent and of parental permission has entered the picture and complicated an already confused situation.

We are often faced with the question of medical treatment and the patient's convenience. The use of home dialysis could conceivably reduce the overall costs of renal dialysis by several billion dollars per year but most patients resist the procedure and physicians do not insist. On the other hand, does the physician have the right to keep a ninety-year-old woman in the hospital because she is more comfortable there or fail to refer a patient from the hospital to a nursing home when the family prefers hospital care even though it is ineffective?

The prevention of disease has been stressed as the ultimate only hope for reducing cost of care. Yet physicians do little about prevention. They have traditionally been willing to provide immunization to children but have not been counselors to the family on the major diseases caused by habits and life styles and have not assumed a major role in education at the lower levels where their presence could make an impact on prevention. Medical direction must take this path. As we eliminate the bacterial infections we are left with the chronic diseases of arthritis, cancer, heart disease, obesity, and mental disorders which we cannot cure with any degree of certainty but which, in many cases, can be alleviated or restrained by preventive measures. It should be remembered that the chronic diseases cost society more in the long run and yet have less done about curing them. It has been suggested that medical care should be provided only to the extent that social benefits equal to or greater than the cost of care are realized from the treatment. It is very apparent that, in many cases, such is not the case and we are spending a great deal on cases which return nothing to society because patients remain incapacitated after treatment, or die.

The physician is faced with a problem in dealing with patients. Although prevention is the only final solution to medical care problems, the patient often resists preventive measures. The average American feels that the environment cannot be controlled and therefore prevention should not be a worry; that the control of smoking or diabetes or obesity interferes with the affluent society; that there is often no concurrence on preventive measures to be taken; and that the role of the consumer in the health care system is ill defined and provides no input into the leaders. Together these factors combine into a potent force to maintain the status quo and thus permit no real changes.

There has been little attempt to control the expenses of the large corporations in providing health care for employees. General Motors has estimated that health care adds $600 to the cost of a car and other companies spend as much as $2,500 per year per employee to provide health care. Here, prevention could make a major impact if the physician participated fully in an educational program.

The control of health care costs have become a major concern of most large companies. The insurance plans of many companies are "cradle to grave" as a result of union pressure and the costs are mounting rapidly. As a result, some 80 consortia have been formed between companies to address the problem and place pressure on unions to accept smaller benefits and to control costs.

The Reagan Administration has also adopted a stance that medical insurance paid by the company is a form of income and should be taxed as any other income. Obviously, unions oppose this measure. However, a case can be made that the relatively affluent middle class is obtaining considerable tax advantages through the insurance route while the old and the poor do not obtain this advantage.

All of the above leads to one conclusion which has been confirmed by Field (1970). The modern physician has become specialty oriented and has lost a multidimensional concept of health as a totality. This leaves the consumer unable to consult with anyone who can provide the overview which is necessary to a broad survey of the health care system and its choices. Partly as a result of this situation, we are spending more and more money to correct diseases which are caused directly by poor social inputs. Field has felt that the physician's role is divided into four parts in dealings with patients. There is a "magical" role which arises because of the incantational approach often used by the physician. There is a "religious" role where the patient is reconciled to a mysterious force which may be attacking, and a "pastoral" role which stems from the need for comfort and support. Finally, there is the "technical" role in which solutions to the problems are arrived at by the physician. All four roles must be met in order to satisfy the patient. Too often in modern day medicine, the last role is paramount and the others are neglected except when they in some way satisfy the ego of the physician. We are all aware of the placebo effect or the use of magic spells in the apparent recovery of the patient and the nontechnical aspects of medical care can serve as an explanation for some of these.

With this introduction we may look at some of the latest statistics which define the relationship between physicians and their patients. Simple division reveals that the average physician has about 4,000 patient visits per year and if the average income of physicians is taken into account, the average charge is about $40.

The number of visits to physicians by patients has remained

relatively constant for about 10 years at 1 billion visits per year. Females have more visits per year than males and non-whites have fewer visits than whites although the differences are decreasing (NCHS, 1983). About 75 percent of the population has more than one visit per year and those patients under seven and over seventy-five have the highest number. Almost 70 percent of all visits were in the doctor's office, 13 percent were in the outpatient clinic and about 0.5 percent were in the home. Twelve percent of all visits (?) were by phone. There has been a slight trend upward in the number of visits per person over the past few years which may be attributable to increase in physician numbers and/or recall policy. Seventy-five percent of all people see a doctor at least once a year but some 13 percent have not seen a doctor in more than 2 years.

The statistics are particularly interesting when compared with the advent of Federal control of many of the health care dollars. The average number of visits per person is about 5 per year in the United States. Families earning less than $5,000 per year had many more visits than families earning over $25,000 per year during the period from 1979 to 1980. Blacks had more visits than whites over the same period. This may be due to greater illness among the two groups which, of course, coincide in many respects, or it may be due to Medicaid availability.

The growth of specialty populations and emphasis is clearly marked. The number of patients visiting a GP (general practitioner) declined from 63 percent to about 47 percent in 1980 while the internist's attraction of patients increased from 5.4 percent to 11 percent in the same period. Pediatricians and ob/gyn specialists maintained about the same percent of visits while all others increased from 17.5 percent to 24.6 percent. About 85 percent of visits were for diagnosis or treatment and of this number, about 51 percent were for chronic conditions.

We have mentioned the plight of the elderly. The group as a whole have about twice as many ailments as the general population. They are more often in the hospital and 75 percent of all persons over sixty-five will spend some time in a nursing home. Despite these indications of need, the physician's attention to geriatric problems are minimal. As we have remarked, physicians receive almost no training in dealing with geriatric patients and this extends into their practice. In addition, nursing homes have not been willing to pay the costs of having a physician on the staff. As Salon (1974) found, the average nursing home does not have great medical input. Only 54 percent have physicians on call and probably about 35 percent have physicians who attend, on a regular basis. About 40 percent of the nursing homes have some form of utilization review and, as a result, there is little relation between charges and related illnesses. On the other hand, many nursing homes have only LVNs on duty most of the time. When a nursing home has RNs on duty the attendance of the physician increases. But even in those homes in which the RNs are employed 24 hours a day, the physician spends less than 1 hour per month per patient. In those homes in which only LVNs are employed the average is 17 minutes per patient per month. Considerable questions can be raised as to whether this represents optimum care for geriatric patients.

*Chapter 10*

# THE PHYSICIAN, COMMUNICATIONS AND TECHNOLOGY*

Communication has helped to revolutionize the health care industry in the past few years. Radio has provided advice to emergency technicians in ambulances, cardiac pacemakers have been remotely monitored, computers have been used for all of the housekeeping functions of the hospital related to financial transactions, and the hospital is slowly turning to automated records particularly for billing Medicare and the insurance companies. The demands of the PSRO for information on physician performance has resulted in computerized transfer of records over considerable distances.

Yet the role of technology in medical communication has not been entirely satisfactory. The communication technologies are all experimental and therefore diverse in nature and not easily compared. The social problems often outweigh the technical difficulties and, as a result, create unusual problems.

In assessing any medical technology, communication or other, several questions must be answered.

*Taken in part from J.H.U. Brown, *Telecommunications on Health Care*, CRC Press, Boca Raton, 1982, with permission.

Can the technology actually help solve the problem?

Is the technology worth developing?

Will the technology cause harm as well as good?

We must also consider that, by its very nature, technology will have an impact on all parts of society: the patient and physician, society, medical care, and the economy.

Communication technology cannot be assessed in the same terms as other medical technology, which is evaluated in terms of the medical problem it will solve. Appraisals of most health care systems seek to answer certain questions. How many people are affected? How will it alter practice? Is it dangerous? The assessment of a health care communication system, however, requires that other types of questions be approached. Is the technology available? Will it alter costs of care? What is the medical efficacy? Will society accept new treatment methods? Will the costs to society be too high in insurance costs and quality of life? Is remote care as satisfactory to the patient and the physician as is face to face treatment?

The health care system, as a whole, must also know: How is the mix of treatment to be changed? How can remote services be evaluated? What are the implications on malpractice, fees, costs of medical practice?

All of medical care is grounded in economics. The economic system must address a variety of questions. What is the cost benefit of communications for the entire economy? What is the cost of a system of telecommunication and where should it be established? How is it to be supported? Who will run it? How will this system affect other communications?

To these problems must be added the additional cost of the system and the *evaluation* of the resulting benefits. There has been much talk about the provision of a telecommunication system to small towns to provide health care to small populations. The health care system has not addressed the questions of access, comfort, economic incentives, status cost, and retention of health practitioners in those locations, although each of them must be answered positively and the final costs considered before a system is inaugurated.

It should be remembered that relatively nontechnical procedures may produce the same benefits in health care, with perhaps smaller costs, by making relatively minor changes in the present delivery system rather than by instituting a total restructuring of health care. There are many approaches to this problem. A phone system may be able to provide service equal to that provided by television, at less cost. Transportation to the doctor may be cheaper than establishing a television link. Dozens of other examples come easily to mind.

Overriding many other considerations may be that of political influence. Many states have strict laws requiring the presence of the physician when service is rendered; these laws effectively prohibit the use of telemedicine. There is concern about privacy of the patient and the threat of open access to records posed by a large communication system. Some states do not permit the use of physician assistants, and over all looms the threat of a malpractice suit when service is provided outside a physician's immediate purview. Many of these practical political problems are being addressed in state legislatures and the Congress. The reactionary attitude of many medical societies, the nurse's demands for status, and the hospitals' need for inpatients also provide resistance to changes which could make telemedicine a useful tool. A hospital with 70 percent occupancy is not likely to encourage remote treatment of potential patients.

A discussion of telemedicine must consider both the sociological and technical aspects of the problem. Ancillary equipment such as fiberoptics, microscopes, and the like can be provided, but a major question is one of utilization and cost-benefit. The average physician feels better about a diagnosis and has less fear of malpractice suits if a full armamentarium of sophisticated equipment can be employed. When such devices are coupled to a transmission system, costs may become extremely high, and the quest here should be for the minimum equipment necessary to produce a desired result—not the maximum available.

Other technical problems may occur. Decisions are now being made as to what intercommunications are necessary for PPOs and DRGs. Should the records of every patient be available wherever that person may be? Should statistical data be assessed on a nationwide basis? The National Center for Health Statistics (NCHS) now accumulates data but does so on a local—to area,

to state, to region, to national—base, with appropriate conden-
sation of information at each step. Is this method sufficient?

When doctors use telecommunication, they do not enhance
their ability to handle a patient, they handle more patients. Statistics indicate that the use of mechanical forms of communication
for exchange between doctor and patient may also increase the
time the doctor must spend with each patient. If, in addition,
the patient load is doubled because of the new access, data indicate that waiting times may increase sixfold. On the other hand,
more patients are seen and patients are seen who would otherwise
not have had medical care.

Another major uncertainty concerns finding the most appropriate kind of technology. Experience in pediatric clinics
suggests that up to 80 percent of all cases can be handled by
Nurse Practitioners (NP) on the telephone (Doerman, 1975).
Would a television system permitting supervision by a physician
improve this response greatly? Under what circumstances can
the nonphysician provide all of the necessary care?

Experience with the Advanced Medical Outpatient System
(AMOS) program in which nonprofessionals conduct triage and
treat patients with the aid of a computer protocol indicates that
80 percent of all cases can be handled in this way. Information
suggests that there is a favorable trade-off of cost to effectiveness
of medical treatment with a telecommunication system but no
data really document this. As the telecommunication system de-
velops and remote patient handling becomes routine, can we rely
on the consumer for greater self-help? Theoretically, the patient
could position him or herself before a television screen, communicate with a Physicians's Assistant (PA) at some distance, and
the PA, in turn, could call into a medical center as necessary.
However, it has been pointed out that problems of billing, malpractice insurance, etc., are enormous in undertaking such an
operation.

## HEALTH CARE

The fact is that too often vast amounts of the information
assembled on patients in the form of records and laboratory data
is redundant and unused in the health care system. The hospital's

answers to the following questions should be important in determination of the data to be collected and utilized:

What form of communication is the best?

What information must be transferred?

What medium is best?

How are decisions to be made using the system and who makes them?

What level of reliability is necessary for the particular job?

What level of fidelity is necessary?

The foregoing suggests that any system of technology must be closely and carefully studied and evaluated to determine if the outcome for the patient has actually been improved. For this reason, it is essential to look at assessment and evaluation of such a system. Among the fundamental questions about the applications of technology are the following:

How many people are affected?—a multimillion-dollar solution proposed for a problem affecting only a few thousand may be in question.

Is the technology an innovation in treatment or does it merely make treatment easier for the physician and harder for the patient?

What is the state of the art?

What are the potential dangers to the patient? What are the effects on quality of life? On confidentiality?

What are the effects of society in terms of costs of care?

Further questions can be posed from the standpoint of the hospital and health care system:

What will be the effect on hospital admissions?

What will be the effect on hospital stays if care can be rendered at home?

What will be the effect on satellite clinics if more care is delivered at home?

*advantages*

On a theoretical basis we could expect telecommunication to permit the delivery of health care in areas where it has not been previously available, to connect tertiary providers to the primary provider system, and to provide the tertiary providers with greater flexibility in handling masses of data flowing in the system. It would be hoped that such a scheme could also redistribute the health providers into the medically undeserved areas and permit the use of paramedics to provide care in noncritical areas of medicine. Finally, telecommunication could help to provide the information base to maintain a better cost/quality ratio, reduce duplication, and fill gaps in the present system of health care.

Carey (1978) has pointed out the practical considerations in implementing a communication system. These include:

> *Proximity*—unless the equipment is near the doctor and patient usage may be decreased.
>
> *Location*—turf considerations are important. Complaints with nearby health personnel are common.
>
> *Normal travel*—users will not go out of the way to use a system.
>
> *Need*—the need must be recognized by the user, not the provider.
>
> *Availability*—repair and technically trained personnel must be available to keep the system operative.
>
> *Comfort*—both physiological and psychological comfort must be provided.
>
> *Security*—primary for the user.
>
> *Involvement* of the users.

Reich (1974) has listed the factors necessary for a successful health care system and the same factors could easily be applied to any technical system.

> Availability—readiness
> Accessibility—closeness

Acceptability—desirable features

Appropriateness—rightness of care

Adaptability—ability to meet changing situations

A-one care—competency

Acceptance by physician and patients must be the critical determining factor in the use of a system. The patients, providers, and the payers must accept the system as it is finally developed if it is to be used for both medical care and administrative purposes.

Patients may be reluctant to accept the system because they are not sure of quality care and privacy. On the other hand, they may accept care by providers using telecommunication because it reduces travel time and cost. Doctors may be reluctant to provide remote care because they anticipate difficulty with diagnosis, with the legal problems, quality of care, and the assessment of the reliability of the system. They may accept the system because of time saving and income enhancement.

The insurers may be reluctant to accept the system because they have no method to assure quality of care provided by non-physician providers, because there are often legal restrictions to the use of PAs, and because the costs may be difficult to determine. The only advantage to this group may be lower costs in the future.

The evaluation of such social decisions may be very inaccurate. For example, patients may use the communication links for medical care because they feel the doctor wishes it, because nothing else is available, or because they are interested in receiving attention, all of which are divorced from health care needs.

It has been mentioned that the telephone may be a satisfactory method of telecommunication in a great number of cases. In general, a television channel is necessary only when the patient or the physician needs reassurance, when there must be feedback from the patient which cannot be obtained from the telephone, or when it is necessary to talk to more than one person at a time on a consultation.

## STANDARDS

In order to achieve order in any medical system and determine the results of treatment it is necessary to have standards. Standards may be of two major types: standards of quality which measure the results of a process, and standards of process which measure the conformity to the average. The latter is the method used on assembly lines and measures the reproducibility of a given procedure. Standards of quality are hard to set and still harder to test.

Standards are set in many ways. The government sets standards when it outlines procedures for Medicaid or Medicare, establishes Occupational Safety and Health Administration (OSHA) guidelines, or sets standards for communication in emergency medical systems. Standards are also set by the individual. Paramedics who work alone must have a standard of performance which has been set by the professional for whom they work, but the standards must be maintained by self-assessment.

Standards set by organizations are of several varieties, each with a different approach to control. *Licensing* sets standards of structure in that anyone who fulfills criteria of education may be licensed. *Accreditation* sets a stronger standard of process in that the organization or person must demonstrate skill or facilities in order to achieve the accreditation. Finally, the measurement of performance by utilization review of services or Professional Standard Review Organization (PSO) sets *standards of outcome*.

Unfortunately, in health systems we are largely setting standards of structure determining the kind of service, the technical input, and the reliability of the product. Until the outcomes are examined in terms of cost benefit to the patient and to the system, we will not have standards which are satisfactory.

In medical care the evaluation of a system is often left to the practitioners. This is reasonable because, after all, they are the ones who will use it. However, they may be asked to make judgments in areas where their expertise is limited. In addition, the feedback in the health care system is usually slow or inadequate so that the evaluation may not be satisfactory even when it is attempted.

In order for evaluation to be successful we must be able to

standardize methods of data handling. The creation of a health care system where records can be transferred from one point to another with complete understanding requires the standardization of tests, records, and many other parts of the system. Any savings of scale can be accomplished only with mass production and this requires definition of a standard product. Computer programs have been written for standardized medical records but, to date, the profession has not seen fit to adopt them. The ICD code which codes diseases in common format is now widely accepted and may become the base for further development as we have already discussed with regard to DRGs.

Problems arise in technology assessment because there are no standard methods, social impacts are hard to measure, it is expensive, and cooperation is hard to obtain in the medical field.

The assessment of technology involves a study of possible alternatives before the event. After the technology is in place, it must be evaluated to see if expectations were fulfilled. Evaluation of technology is usually based on three modes (see Fig. 6, page 146):

> *Structure*—the measurement of the physical properties of the system. Did the radios perform as desired? Could the x-ray be read by transmission?
>
> *Process*—the measurement of the variables in the system. Were more patients seen? Was the diagnosis equally good in two different situations of care (television and personal contact)?
>
> *Outcome*—the measurement of a direct effect on health. Did more patients live? Were they in better health?

Obviously, the outcome is the desired measure and the one most difficult to evaluate. There is little agreement about the health outcomes of a given approach to health care and it may be difficult to evaluate the value of communications in the process.

The chain of consultations is shown in Figure 8. This figure illustrates the wide variety of communications which must be established in order effectively to manage a system. Telecommun-

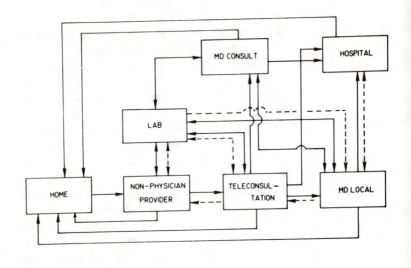

___ PATIENT FLOW
--- TELECOMMUNICATIONS FEEDBACK

**Figure 8.** The flow of patients and information in the doctor's office and into the health care system (from Brown, J.H.U., *Telecommunications in Health Care*, Boca Raton: CRC Press, 1982, with permission).

ication could conceivably be used to link any or all parts of the system and, of course, many of the parts are already linked by telephone at the present time. The many points where evaluation are necessary are obvious.

## THE USE OF COMMUNICATIONS

When single applications of communication are surveyed they can usually be categorized under transmission of visual signal (x-rays), electrical signals (EKG), data (clinical laboratory output) or physical signs (swelling, edema, etc.), and visual display (microscopic slides). In another order of complexity is the transmission of information which allows the physician to make judgments about state of mind (psychiatric interview). Each form of medical data demands a different degree of fidelity and perhaps a different mode of communication (television vs. telephone).

Many of the methods discussed are easy to incorporate into large systems. While it is difficult to get away from the patient-doctor relationship, it is simple for a computer to read x-rays or EKGs transmitted from many locations to a central analytical system and to return the results to the proper location. This, of course, raises the basic question of how the system will be structured. Should there be one network for patient records and one for administrative data, which can be mixed as desired in the clinic or doctor's office? Will one network carry all necessary information? Again, the precision of transmitted medical or laboratory information and the use the physician makes of such information is quite different from the accuracy of information which the physician will accept in dealing directly with a patient. Examination of a slide or an x-ray picture does not place the physician in a peer review mode with colleagues nor raise serious questions of malpractice as does the direct patient contact.

It is difficult to separate the role of the computer from that of telecommunication. The computer may be online but at a remote distance from the parameter under measurement. As a result, many of the functions which are computer controlled also are remote operations. We have chosen to list some of these functions in generic terms with the understanding that there are many other examples.

Projects in telecommunication for primary health care delivery have usually been set up to demonstrate one or more of the modes of operation of a clinic. They have all suffered from a few common troublesome traits.

The transmission of medical material, ranging from handwritten medical records through typed material to radiographs, has presented technical problems, including those of resolution.

Two points can be made about this particular application. First, the electrocardiogram is a narrowband physiological signal for which television transmission is bandwidth wasteful and costly. In this case it is obvious (because telephone-based EKG systems already exist) that there is a cost-effective way to transmit the information that is required. In other cases, where different kinds of signals are sent, this may not be as obvious. For example, the transmission of handwritten records and typed material requires superior resolution. The use of the standard phone line transmission system to teletype documents (QWIP) has not been widely adopted although it could again decrease the bandwith needed.

The telephone is the most important telecommunication device. Television may also be important but, in many cases, it can be used as a confirmation rather than to secure primary information. However, some problems remain. There is wide disagreement about the value of some forms of television. We have already mentioned the wastefulness of using television to transmit EKGs on a broadband channel. Secondly, some groups believe that x-rays read by television are as satisfactory as those read in person, but others have found that the radiologists must see more views of the x-ray over a television channel in order to make a diagnosis.

The highest resolution required for graphics in health care may be for the transmission of radiographs. The radiologist may have to request several successive views of close-ups of the film to make a diagnosis and thus must wait while the technician or general practitioner on site adjusts the camera to the specific area the radiologist wants to see better. These procedures make x-ray viewing by television a very time-consuming procedure. New methods must be developed.

The ability to read charts over a television channel has not yet been well developed and it may, in fact, prove to be better to send the chart from one location to another by the usual telephone data transmission system as opposed to sending the chart intact to be read from a cathode ray tube. Further improvement in the patient record should also be explored. It is possible to produce abstracts of the record which are satisfactory and can be used in a remote location rather than transmitting the entire, bulky, redundant, and often erroneous record over a television channel.

A legally valid signature is required on certain medical documents (e.g., hospital admission slip, prescriptions, doctors' orders, and hospital discharge summary). An original signature implies personal presence and, presumably, cognizance of the document being signed, so that responsibility rests unambiguously with the signing individual. Our medical care system is firmly grounded on this principle. Electrowriters have been used to transmit signatures, but this technique introduces its own problem because once the signature is electronically transmittable it is electronically reproducible and the personal responsibility concept is jeopardized.

As pointed out in Bashur (1977), evaluation of a project may require measurement of such items as:

Cost/benefit
Privacy
Responsibility
Compatibility with existing systems of care
Flexibility

Unfortunately, all of these items are either structural or process in nature and do not deal with whether the patient has actually benefited at less cost or with greater access.

It is obvious to the economist and the operations research expert that the problems of medicine are much the same as other problems of economics. The parameters of measurement are different, but the final results must be expressed in terms of cost benefit, outcomes, and other similar evaluation parameters. As with many other facets of medical economy, not much is known about the elasticity of the system or the response to aggregation to larger units to reduce costs. All of these problems must be investigated.

## TECHNOLOGY IN HEALTH CARE

In any network, medical or other, we must look first at the linkages. Communications is the major link in health care. Communicators may be linked to a physician and a patient through a computer, direct contact, ancillary equipment (x-ray reader, EKG reader, etc.) or an intermediary (dispatcher, etc.). In addition to the communication links, a medical input must also be present. If health care is to be given at a remote site, it is essential for a protocol of treatment to be developed which will clearly define responsibility, provide a framework for decision making, and establish a means for the physician to be assured that orders are being followed. In order to perform such tasks the protocol must address such questions as the following:

What are the goals of the system?
What kind of health problems are addressed?
What kind of providers will be used?
How will the system be evaluated?

Results are often the best obtainable but not necessarily the most desirable. The use of telemedicine may permit more patients to be seen, but as the contact time decreases, the quality of care may also decrease. The cost of the system may be high, but it may be a trade-off from long travel times or no care at all.

Any system of communication must be able to handle a medical problem in the same way a physician handles it. The accuracy with which care is delivered and disease diagnosed, the number of repeat analyses necessary to obtain the desired information, the time required, and the relationship of the patient to the system are all influences on acceptance of a communications system. When a system is adopted, the establishment of new stages in medical care is required. Except for the treatment in the office of local specialists, the system may depend upon the development of a system of integrated primary care because of the difficulty of connecting many physicians into a network to treat the single patient. The use of paramedical personnel in some form to perform the basic services will require a location where communication can be established and maintained.

This is not the place to discuss the role of the nonphysician provider. Suffice it to say that the communications system should assist the pretreatment work-up plus treatment of cases under remote supervision and follow-up or handling cases where the physician is not needed. Description of protocols for such methods have been provided by Doerman (1975).

It has been remarked that a doctor has attributes which enable him or her to practice medicine effectively. These are reliability, sustenance (reassurance), and a variety of omnipotence. It is doubtful that communication and the paramedic can effectively replace all of these, although, in some cases reliability, the system may actually outperform the physician.

Another major problem affecting the communication between doctor and patient is the attitude of the provider. A summary of these problems would include: (1) dislike of waiting, (2) failure to listen, and (3) failure to explain—all of which are aggravated by telecommunication. On the other hand, doctors also dislike house calls and they are easily bored by routine, both of which may be partly alleviated by communication. Physicians are also bored by frequent patient visits about minor ills and about long discussion of minor illness, both of which can be reduced by the proper use of telemedicine.

Some attention should be given to the psychological requirements of telemedicine. Thus, it has been suggested that in an augmented verbal communication between a physician and patient, it may be more important for the patient to be able to view the physician than for the physician to be able to view the patient. The potential of videotaping for this purpose is still largely untapped. Data indicate that video consultations take twice as long on the average as do telephone consultations and taping may be a solution to this problem because the physician can review the data at leisure.

Television affects only some of the senses upon which we rely for information input into the brain. Sight and sound are available in telecommunications but we are unable to use taste, smell, touch, heat, proximity, and eye contact—all of which are important in our overall communication scheme.

It may well be that we will eventually find that many of these inputs are essential for full communication. However, to date, experience of Americans (black and white), American Indians, Aleuts (Eskimos), Eastern Indians, and Japanese indicates that the handicap is not great.

However, it is true that with each loss of sense the physician loses an input to judgment. Many physicians correct for the loss by requesting additional tests or by spending more time with the patient. Both procedures increase the overall costs of care. This general statement has been questioned by Conroth (1974) who found the contrary, that deprivation of modes of sensory input had very little effect on time spent with the patient or on the final diagnosis.

An interesting relationship exists between referrals of a patient from a paramedic to the physician and the use of telecommunication. The referral proved to be related to the disease and not to the use of the telephone. In those cases in which a decision could be reached easily over the phone, the percentage of referrals decreased markedly. In the more difficult cases, or those cases in which telephone conversation did not provide the information necessary to reach a decision, the extent of referrals greatly increased (Bashur, 1977). For example, with ear problems, upper respiratory infections, and GI problems, the referrals were reduced about 20 percent. The referrals for obstetrics and gynecology cases were reduced only 5 percent. The reasons are apparent.

The communication system requirements for terminal location and the associated requirements for terminal ubiquity, point-to-point switching capability, and terminal portability have proven to be unexpectedly difficult to define. Their definition is likely to require particularly sensitive interaction between the engineers and the health care system planners.

The cost calculations must go beyond the direct hardware and personnel costs. For example, the effect of video vs. telephone consults on the error rates of referrals and their associated costs, i.e., the cost of an unnecessary referral and the cost of failing to refer when a referral is indicated, has not been determined. There may be hidden social costs, e.g., time lost from work, costs borne by the patient, hire of babysitters for an unnecessary referral, or by increased morbidity for the missed referral, in which case it would be difficult to measure dollar savings which are directly applicable to the communication system. However, if the health care system pays for transportation, or must send consultants to the patient, then the costs might be convertible from one system to the other.

In addition, the requirements for visual telecommunication might profitably be studied from the perspective of an integrated communication system permitting audio, video, and digital information transmission. Medical information systems for patient care, administration, auditing, and other functions are already under development. Since the hardware can be used for multiple function, it is reasonable to anticipate that an integrated, multipurpose communication system whose hardware costs are spread over these several functions could be economically attractive, though a system designed for only one of the functions might remain unattractive.

The institutional, organizational, and other constraints that will affect the prospect of visual telecommunications as an innovation will have to be identified. For example, there are few precedents for reimbursing physicians for teleconsults, or for paying nonphysicians for services provided when not under the (in-person) supervision of a physician. Without some kind of incentive, the prospects are dim for widespread adoption even assuming that careful research has demonstrated that certain health care functions can be effectively and efficiently performed with such innovations.

There may also be a resistance to change, or at least a lack of incentive for change, on the part of individuals who do not benefit directly from the telecommunication innovation. For example, one reason suggested for the low level of utilization of telecommunication by physicians was that the major benefits accrued to patients, not physicians. Travel has already been reduced to a near minimum by various means, such as use of hospital space and the location of offices near hospitals. Thus, there is little incentive for the physicians to unlearn their accustomed ways of accomplishing a task and suffer through the inefficiencies and frustrations associated with learning a task in a new (and eventually better) way.

Patient care includes diagnosis and therapy and follow-up visits. Experience suggests that telemedicine may decrease physician "productivity" because a patient visit over television may take longer than an in-person visit, while yielding benefits such as saving patient's travel. This illustrates the conflicting performance goals of the health care system; in this case, a benefit from the patient's point of view is a cost from the provider's point of view. We must eventually decide on a total cost-benefit ratio by a close evaluation of the system. However, several workers appear to agree that the number of referrals is reduced through the use of telecommunication. Doerman and co-workers (1978) found that the referrals could be reduced 25 percent with the use of the telephone and about 60 percent when television was used as the communication link.

As medical costs continue to increase, it is apparent that new methods of long-term care outside the hospital or nursing home must be adopted. Experiments are proceeding in several directions. Two obvious methods can be used—prevention and self-care.

The high cost of the physician in delivery of health care has generated considerable thought toward the development of alternative methods of providing care. The PA is challenging the belief that only physicians can carry out certain tasks related to patient care. Only a few PAs have been graduated, but some 80 programs exist, and some 50 others are studying the role of the NP in this area. The AMOSISTS Program of the Army uses medics to treat more than 50 percent of all outpatients in a major hospital, using a computer-driven telecommunications system. The use of physicians in the New York City School System has decreased markedly; the physicians have been replaced by NPs at about half the costs.

Major questions have arisen concerning the use of paramedical personnel of whatever type. Remotely situated paramedics come under a dual suspicion; they are suspected of not calling the doctor when it is necessary, thus providing inadequate medical care, but, on the other hand, they may be forced to perform tasks beyond their capability because of inadequate supervision by the remote doctor. Both problems have been raised as serious objection to the use of PAs or NPs. Studies conducted by Ekwo (1979) have indicated that this is not a serious problem and that, in his studies, the physician was actually consulted in all life-threatening cases. Ross (1973) has examined the physician's role in delivery of remote health care and found that the discontinuity of care resulting from remote contact, or from several physicians consulting with the same patient over a period of time, was not serious and resulted in no clearcut relationship between telecommunication methods and the quality of care given. They report that the greatest possibility of error might be some omissions in treatment or diagnosis resulting from infrequent contact between patient and physician.

The use of the PA appeals to economists and politicians for several reasons. It would help alleviate the MD shortage (if one exists) at a reduced cost, it would employ additional skills, and it would save money. It may also provide better overall health care because in rural areas where there are no physicians the PA can be certified to perform many of the duties of a physician, including physical exams, minor surgery, and other procedures.

The Cambridge Project has a computer program to compare costs of the physician vs. costs of a paramedic working with a communications system. They conclude the PA is 20 percent less effective than the MD but this does not take into account the fact that one MD may have two or more PAs working under his or her direction, while, at the same time, the MD is conducting a regular practice. Expenses cannot be compared between operating systems because costs depend so much on local variables that it is difficult to assign accurate costs. Many systems are not cost effective because of unnecessary equipment or because the system handles too few patients. Present evidence is that a single frame black and white TV and phone may serve as well as more complicated systems, and would materially reduce costs.

The major problem concerning acceptance of the PA for health care delivery has been sociological in nature. It has been expressed in resistance by the nurses as a response to the development of the PA. The PA often takes second place only to the MD and the nurse. The American Medical Association (AMA), as long ago as 1966, invited the American Nursing Association (ANA) to develop programs to make the nurse a PA. Instead the nursing schools elected to offer a PhD in nursing and to create the NP.

The American Academy of Pediatrics has also tried to enlist the NAs in pediatric practice with the same rebuff. The nurses make it very clear that "the question is not who does what, but who prescribes and who delegates to whom."

## THE ELDERLY

A major field for telecommunication is in the nursing homes. This project is of particular importance because recent surveys (1982) indicate that only 36 percent of nursing homes have regular physician visits. Only 54 percent have physicians on call; 40 percent have no utilization review and physicians spend only from 17 to 68 min/patient/month in giving care to nursing home residents. Telecommunications can provide the vital link in the system because nursing home residents use three times the amount of medical services used by the average American.

There is another aspect of the care of the elderly where telecommunications offers major advantage. It has been discovered that, in many cases, the elderly do better when left at home as opposed to being placed in a hospital or nursing home. However, such procedure requires some means of contact with the patient on a regular basis and some form of alerting system must be available when the patient needs immediate care. The development of an alert system for the blind, which can call a special number without their dialing, is a case in point. An obvious advantage would be an interactive television system but this is probably beyond the cost range of most health systems at the present time.

In order partially to investigate this problem, New York University has set up an interactive cable system in Reading, Pa. to provide communications to the elderly (Marshall, 1977). Because of expense, the links were not to individual homes. Rather, three centers, including two senior citizens' housing projects, were linked and converters were installed in the homes of the elderly so they could watch but not participate in interactions. Interactions included social service, public service, health, amusement, and development of new skills. The total cost was about $100,000/ year. The basic principles in operation of the system were use of senior citizens as initiators, use of local facilities, reliance on spontaneous programs, and the emphasis on programming to serve special groups such as the elderly. This is not an expensive system and it may lead to development of cost effective systems in the future.

## RURAL HEALTH

Rural health care is a serious problem. Infant mortality is greater in rural areas. More accidents occur in rural areas and the death rate is 66 percent higher for workers in rural industry than for other industrial employees (1982). Limitations due to chronic conditions are 30 percent greater on the farm than in urban areas. As the average age of farm workers increases, as it has for the past 2 decades, the limitation of chronic conditions must also increase. The number of farm workers who have been screened for cancer and heart disease is less than for other elements of the population.

The problem is complicated by the lack of professional personnel. There has been a continual decrease in the number of physicians in rural areas. There are now about 71 physicians per 100,000 rural population as compared to 151 physicians per 100,000 population in metropolitan areas (Anon, 1982). The lack of specialists is a major problem. The best estimates are that 131 physicians per 100,000 population are needed to provide adequate medical attention. Even if a lower figure, such as that used by Kaiser Foundation (80 physicians per 100,000) is adopted, there are 21,000,000 rural residents in 60 percent of the nation's counties whose health care needs must now be met with lower ratios (Anon, 1982).

The simple ratio is a reflection of the quantity but not of the quality of health care. Factors must be weighted by the milieu in which practice occurs. Productivity is often decreased by transportation problems and poorer hospital facilities, despite the fact that the rural doctor may see more patients per day than the urban practitioner. Quality may also be decreased in rural areas. The average age of physicians is considerably greater in rural than in urban America, few physicians are Board Certified, and few appear to keep up with medical advances. The rural physician also faces a greater need. The population is less affluent, is engaged in more hazardous occupations, is older, and is less educated in rural America.

The few experiments on the use of telecommunications in rural health care suggest that the role of nonphysician health workers can be expanded, the number of referrals can be decreased, and that relatively low level technology (telephone) can suffice in many instances. The use of the telephone alone to provide consultation to the NP or rural physician decreases referrals 25 percent (Bashur, 1976). Protocols devised to make use of telecommunications on the Navajo Indian Reservation resulted in referral of patients to the physician 29 percent of the time, whereas an equivalent population without technology were referred 58 percent of the time. As could be expected, the percentage of referred patients varied with condition, ob-gyn being referred very often while patients with cuts, bruises, etc. were seldom referred.

The political problems accompanying provisions of primary care in rural areas are critical. A few simple examples illustrate the point. If tax moneys are used in rural areas, how should funds be provided? On a per capita basis the rural areas will get little care because of the costs of transportation and services. If the funding is on the basis of health care costs, rural areas will receive much greater funds per capita than urban areas because of expenses. The extent of services provided are usually less in rural than in urban areas regardless of funding. It is difficult to recruit, train, and maintain manpower. Hospitals are often small and not well equipped, and sophisticated procedures are often not available. Each of these problems suggests the need for a better system.

## THE AUTOMATED PHYSICIAN'S ASSISTANT

The Automated Physician's Assistant (APA) (Bass, 1972) is a computer-oriented system designed to increase efficiency of the solo practitioner in remote areas by providing otherwise unobtainable information and services and full communications with a university medical center. In the APA system, the patient operates a terminal in the physician's office and enters data concerning personal medical history. In addition to the automated patient history, a number of other functional computer program packages tailored to the needs of the rural practicing physician have been developed. These programs permit patient data from the physician's office to be entered into a large central computer at a remote location. Patient data consist of vital signs, hearing test results (audiometer), vision test results (acuity, phoria, color perception, etc.) and reports on x-ray, blood chemistry analysis, urine analysis, hematology, pulmonary function, physical examination findings, diagnosis, and treatment or therapy.

Programs have been developed which display upon the office terminal various reports pertaining to a particular patient, which can be called up quickly for review by the physician. Another program has the capability of inserting, deleting, or modifying an entry to update or correct files. At present, blood samples from the physician's office are transported to automatic analyzers. The results of these tests are entered into the patient's file via terminals located in the pathology laboratory. The physician has access to this information as soon as the entry has been made from the pathology laboratory. Blood chemistry and hematology data are also available from the physician's office.

A summary of all of the information available about a particular patient can be obtained from a printer located in the physician's office. The summary report includes all the medical data such as the patient history; the specialized reports of pathology, radiology, EKG, etc., the diagnosis, and the treatment plan prescribed to the patient. The patient's history, the vital signs, vision and hearing tests, EKG interpretation, urinalysis report, the x-ray report, and pulmonary function test results can be made available to the physician before the physical examination is given. The physical examination results, clinical impressions, and the treatment prescribed are also entered.

An EKG recorded signal is transmitted to an automatic tape recorder, converted to digital form, and analyzed by a program in the central computer. Results are entered directly into the patient file with the other information. The results are available to the physician for display or for hard copy printout as soon as they are entered into the file.

All of the programming and the information processing and reporting programs are in daily use in the office of Dr. B.J. Bass during the normal operating day. Dr. Bass is a general practitioner based in a very rural area near Salem, Missouri. He uses the APA in a flexible manner, using the functions provided by the system which are most appropriate for the individual patient being seen. This experiment thus far has been aimed at development of computer-based aids for care in ambulatory settings. The program has developed and tested various components of computer-based ambulatory care measurement devices as well as ambulatory care information systems.

Major issues must be examined before we can conclude that technological components are effective in rural health care delivery systems, and can, in truth, be cost effective and accepted by the health care community. In addition to the usual concerns of quality and quantity of care, a serious question for the APA is the cost per patient if the device were to be widely used by the solo physician.

## SOME APPLICATIONS

Many attempts have been made to read x-rays by computer or by transmission of the x-ray to a remotely situated radiologist. Despite the recurrent data indicating that too many x-rays are taken unnecessarily, there are still large areas of the country where no radiologist is available at all. In many cases a radiology department in a small hospital urgently needs to consult with a specialist. Ward rounds can be conducted remotely without the need of handling large bulky films if the films are available on television monitors. For these reasons, attempts have been made since 1966 to read radiographs remotely.

Part of the problem in the use of remote radiology techniques has been that radiologists must learn a new method of scanning films when they are projected. There are differences in contrast and intensity which can be compensated, in part, by the zoom lens of the television camera. However, once this minor problem has been overcome, the accuracy is high. Pictures of x-rays have been transmitted for several years to the Massachusetts General Hospital Emergency Room from a television emergency system at Boston's Logan Airport. Diagnoses were made solely from the film. Murphy (1970) found that 92 percent of films remotely read agreed with the diagnosis of a panel of experts. In fact, there was some tendency to "over-read"—to read more into a film than was actually present. Some of the radiologists preferred an 825-line system giving a finer resolution but the standard 525-line system appears to be equally good.

Telecommunications are also used to plan radiation treatments, using a computer program to define placement of radiation. The Biomedical Engineering Center at Washington University in St. Louis, Missouri has a variety of treatment programs on the computer which can be transmitted to various locations. The radiologist decides on intensity and areas to be protected and the computer prepares a treatment plan.

Slack and Van Cura (1968) have also developed a computer protocol for determining treatment of patients. The patients indicate answers to a series of questions posed by computer arranged in a decision tree designed to provide diagnosis for allergic reactions. The nonallergic patient may answer 15 questions while the allergic patient may answer 500 to increase accuracy of the diagnosis. The accuracy of diagnosis is very high, and both patients and doctors are satisfied. The same authors have developed a protocol for gastrointestinal problems similar to the allergy plan described above. In their experience, patients appear to enjoy themselves. The patients prefer the computer to the physician in general medical problems, but have a slight preference for the doctor in specialized conditions.

Wittson and Benshote have described a two-way television system which links the University of Nebraska Medical Center to the Norfolk Mental Hospital, 112 miles away. The system has been used for patient consultation, ward control, administration, and education. It provides a neurologist to read electroencephalograms (EEGs) and enables three psychiatrists at the medical center to deal with 10 wards at the hospital. Three VA hospitals are now in the circuit. The system operates about 68 percent of the time for administration and 25 percent for patient care. Costs are about $5/hr for rented lines. Many of the staff are not totally happy with the methodology because of the lack of "hands-on" medicine.

Straker and Mostzen operate a television system between Mount Sinai Medical School and Wagner Child Health Clinic, with two NPs, and found much the same reaction. There was little or no objection on the part of patients or parents. In fact, the authors found that patients accepted the consultation better when presented on television than when they were forced to travel to meet the psychiatrist in person in unfamiliar surroundings. The authors also videotaped conferences and cases for staff review and found them to be very useful for education of staff.

The use of telecommunication for diagnosis in dermatology has been tested with the unit which has been in operation for some 10 years between Logan Airport and Massachusetts General Hospital. A careful study revealed that a high percentage of correct diagnoses could be made remotely. In the experiment, color and black and white slides were read by a dermatologist and by an internist not trained in dermatology but who occasionally saw such patients. The study revealed that technical expertise in the television system was critical. Focusing and contact were both important. Of greater interest was the finding that black and white TV was almost as effective as color in making the diagnosis and that both were about as effective as direct vision. Other reports stress the value of color TV in some dermatological diagnosis.

At the present time, millions of EKGs are being read over various links to computers from doctor's offices and hospitals. Since the first EKG was read by computer in 1969, the practice has become a viable commercial enterprise. At the present time, in locations of high volume, EKGs can be read for less than $2 each, with an accuracy of about 90 percent depending on the desired interpretation and the number of parameters evaluated. Differences of interpretation occur between cardiologists much of the time and this error is not considered excessive.

State University of New York Medical Center, Kings County Hospital, has a phonecomputer link which asks 122 questions of patients submitting to neurological screening. The interviews, administered by protocol, were supervised by medical students and a Registered Nurse (RN). About 75 percent of the computer referrals were found to be appropriate as were 86 percent of the computer-determined patient discharges. Only 10 percent of the patients were dissatisfied with the procedure.

Several pharmacy protocols have been developed where patient data are entered into the pharmacy terminal and a remote computer makes checks on the correct dose, determines compatibility of drugs ordered, prints labels, gives stop orders for drugs, schedules drugs, provides a medication chart for each patient, and bills the patient.

Interpretation of heart sounds is an important diagnostic technique. The Logan Airport-MGH System has been used for some time to transmit heart sounds and phonograms. All heart sounds except for the faintest of murmurs can be easily read over the microwave link or heard over the audio circuits. Phonograms are said to be identical between the radio link and in the physician's office. In a test on consecutive patients there were no false positives or negatives and only minor disagreement in grade of heart murmurs.

It is possible to monitor and treat the desperately ill patient by making an initial assessment of status, initiating protocols for therapy, determining metabolic balance and renal function, and automatically controlling fluid and other intake remotely. A variety of systems for remote monitoring or metabolic function have been developed including those at Columbia University College of Physicians and Surgeons, University of Buffalo, and elsewhere. The system is an extension of the Intensive Care Unit (ICU) monitoring used in many hospitals but it monitors and controls more parameters.

A critical problem in most medical systems is the extent of adverse drug reactions. Sweden has an extensive network to monitor drug reactions. Lemuel Shuttuck Hospital in Boston has been monitoring drug reactions for some time. The communication system is largely computer oriented and is designed to flag reactions and drugs. In 830 patients there were 405 drug reactions of which 25 percent were considered severe (Cohen, 1972). Most of the reactions were due to iatrogenic problems, i.e., interaction between drugs prescribed by the physician rather than patient idiosyncrasy.

Personnel trained in poison information, in handling poison cases, and in a proper referral of such cases, are vital to the emergency system of any large city. Experiences in the San Diego Poison Center, which is one of the best in the country, indicate that the establishment of a good poison control center resulted in an increase in the number of calls in 1 year from approximately 6,800 to more than 18,000. The poison control center is also a means of reducing the cost of medical care. It has been reliably estimated that a 40 percent reduction in poison cases admitted to the hospital can occur with a good poison control center which can provide home remedies and advice by phone on poison cases. This reduction in poison cases admitted to the hospital results in savings of approximately $2 million/year in hospital costs at a cost of less than $4/call. The poison centers in Denver, Galveston, and Kansas City, as well as in San Diego, operate on a national and even international basis, often using computerized files.

# Chapter 11

# A SUMMING UP

The mores of American medicine are changing. The change has come about because of the emergency need for better management and for tighter controls on quality of care within the doctor's office and within the system. This has occurred for several reasons.

The shift in ownership of hospital beds has had an influence. Today, one out of every three beds belongs to a chain of hospitals and one out of eight beds belongs to a for-profit operation. Both the chains and, in particular, the for-profit hospitals are concerned with better management and control of health care delivery. This has worked in two directions. In the first place, the for-profit chains have insisted on control of purchasing and ordering of materials and on the use of technology unless it is clearly profitable. On the other hand, the desire to make a profit has made the for-profits encourage the physicians to use available technology to the limit especially with regard to laboratory tests and procedures.

About 10 percent of all hospitals (1,050) were owned by for-profit organizations in 1982 and another 4 percent were under management of for-profit companies. One corporation (HCA) owns about 5 percent of all beds in the country. Hospitals are not the only source of profits. About 75 percent of all nursing homes are privately owned as are some 40 percent of all kidney dialysis centers. There are some 600 "ambulatory care centers" and centers of many other types including clinical testing, dental care, weight control, and a variety of others.

Interestingly enough, the for-profit hospitals have many more physicians on their board than the voluntary hospitals. In some 60 percent of for-profit hospitals physicians are the board majority. This raises questions about conflict of interest, profit sharing, and similar charges (Gray, 1983).

Another influence has been the increase in group practice. Now more than 25 percent of all physicians are in some group as compared with a negligible number 20 years ago. In addition, most young medical graduates are finding that it is imperative to enter a group in order to develop a practice without the enormous front end expense now necessary to equip an office. In some respects this provides the patient with better care because there are specialists under the same roof readily available. On the other hand, it is more expensive care because every member of the group is a specialist and charges accordingly.

There has been a shift in the general overview of medicine as seen by its practitioners. We entered a phase of medical practice and specialization after World War II which developed the specialist system. In the 1960s medicine entered a planning phase in an attempt to organize and control the system. Now, as the number of beds and physicians increases, the trend is to develop market strategies to sell a product.

There are mounting pressures from the consumer. It has not been too many years ago that the doctor was considered to be an omnipotent healer who was listened to with deference. The high costs of medical care now lead to a questioning of that attitude and the development of new systems of care. Canada developed a system of National Health Care. The United States has not yet reached that point. However, we are seeing the rise of the Health Maintenance Organization and the PPO as the alternative. HMOs and PPOs, with their prospective payment systems, have been the first break in the long chain of higher hospital costs and more expensive medicine.

We are just beginning to realize that we are paying a tremendous overhead for an antiquated system which does not provide the service needed. The development of the marketing strategies mentioned above has led to the development of hospital ambulatory care clinics with the high costs of hospital facilities whose only real function is to fill hospital beds.

On the other hand, we are seeing the rise of stand-alone clinics, one-day surgeries, and other similar care systems designed to make a profit for the owner but providing care at a more reasonable cost to the consumer.

In the development of a method of provision of health care we have not developed a system. The physician and the hospital stand alone but are, of course, closely interrelated. However, neither is related to the nursing home, outpatient facilities, home care, or preventive medicine. No real system of progression depending upon the type or degree of illness exists. This is the reason that 80 percent of desperately ill people die in the hospital when many of them could die more easily in a hospice or at home. Fortunately we are beginning to see the rise of the hospice movement in the United States.

We have made medical care too easy to obtain and too cheap for the consumers because they do not pay the direct costs except through a third party. The third party reimbursement system has tended to separate the consumer from the costs of care and has resulted in a system of expensive, hard-to-justify care. The tendency of the Federal government to increase copayments in its programs is probably a step in the right direction.

Although we blame the hospital for the increasing costs of medical care, we must ultimately realize that it is the physician who places the patient in the hospital, orders the many tests given, and determines the length of stay. The implementation of UR and PSRO may eventually tend to restrict this privilege and contain the excesses, but we have not yet reached the point where mature decisions are made on the questions of costs and benefit.

Perhaps unfortunately, the physician is human. He or she tends to follow the latest trends in medicine and give the latest drugs touted by the sales representatives without due consideration of the costs or the final outcome. We have focussed on the outcomes of medicine—did the patient actually leave the system better off than when he or she entered it—measured by overall health, not only today but in the future. Questions are now being raised about the use of surgery, excessive prescribing of drugs, and the use of testing procedures which may be worse than the disease.

As the cost of medical care rises toward one trillion dollars per year and more than 10 percent of the Gross National Product, many of the topics are coming to a head in the attempts to control the economics of health care. Federal legislation is already addressing some of the issues but many more need to be carefully examined.

Some 23,000,000 Americans have high blood pressure. We must come eventually to a means of monitoring the least critically ill of these and provide treatment in the home. The same situation obtains with other chronic illnesses. The diabetic can be trained to regulate blood sugar and diet. The Bolt, Baranek, and Newman CAPO computer-assisted training operation currently furnishes patient education programs in diabetes, family planning, obesity, lung disease, dieting, and hypertension. The several programs now available to allow patients to take their own medical history in a computer format offer a similar opportunity.

The physician should be more concerned about personal relationships with patients. A survey made in 1978 by the Robert Wood Johnson Foundation found that 61 percent of people believed that a crisis existed in health care; 29 percent of those tested believed that they knew more about their own health than the doctor; that it is very difficult to get admitted to a hospital without proof of ability to pay (56 percent); 40 percent believe that doctors fail to explain enough to patients; 48 percent thought that medical care could be better; and 51 percent thought that family doctors were in very short supply. On the other hand, some 84 percent of those tested were willing to accept medical care from nurse practitioners.

Together this reflects a picture of a certain lack of confidence in the system and a need to modify approaches to the delivery of care.

The hospital and the physician have a tendency to claim that the health care system in the United States is the best in the world. This clearly reflects the marketing aspects. There is no question but that we have the most expensive system in the world for value received but there is considerable question as to whether we have the best system in the world. In part the matter is a question of definition. If the definition rests upon the most expensive gadgets and the largest number of operations, we have the best system. If it rests upon equal care for the whole population, reasonable costs, and satisfactory outcomes, we are far from having the best system. Dr. John Knowles (1978) summed up the problem in the title of his book: *Doing Better and Feeling Worse*.

The health care system and the consumer must face the fact that there is no excuse for a system in which the costs of care rise faster than the cost of living or the GNP. Eventually the decision will have to be made as to how much of the GNP the taxpayer is willing to devote to health care. There are already signs of discontent. Unless the medical profession is able to demonstrate a greater cost benefit for the technology costs in health care, such care will rapidly become too expensive. The demand for costly procedures such as transplantations are bound to increase but we are likely to be forced into a situation where some means other than the taxpayer or the general hospital population will be expected to pay for them. The inequity of the situation becomes more and more apparent as we expend larger sums on the individual patient and therefore, by necessity, less on the average user of the system.

We must change the system from a "sick care" to a "health care" management operation with the introduction of better preventive measures, better environmental analysis, and better patient education.

# BIBLIOGRAPHY

Abayoni, D. Value of routine tests for evaluation of gynecologic malignancy. *Biophy*, 1982, *8*, 24.

Abdellah, F. The nurse practitioner 17 years later. *Inquiry*, 1982, *19*, 105.

Abel-Smith, B. *Money for value in health services*. New York: St. Martins Press, 1976.

Andersen, R., Kravits, J., & Andersen, O. W. *Equity in health services*. Cambridge, Ma.: Ballinger Press, 1975.

Applegate, W. B., Bennett, M. D., Chilton, L., Skipper, B. J., & White, R. E. Impact of a cost containment educational policy in clinic charges. *Medical Care*, 1983, *21*, 48.

Attinger, E., & Theodordis, G. C. Engineering approaches to societal systems. In J. H. U. Brown & J. F. Dickson, *Advances in biomedical engineering* (Vol. 5). New York: Academic Press, 1975.

Bailey, R. M. From professional monopoly to corporate oligarchy. *Medical Care*, 1977, *15*, 129.

Barda, I. T., Sloan, D., & Jick, H. Assessment of adverse drug reactions in a drug surveillance program. *J.A.M.A.*, 1968, *205*, 645.

Barry, V. *Moral aspects of health care*. Belmont, Ca.: Wodsworth Press, 1982.

Barzel, Y. Costs of medical treatment, 1968, *American Educator 58*, 93T.

Bashur, R., & J. Lovett. An assessment of telemedicine. *Advances in Space and Environmental Medicine*, 1977, *48*, 65.

Bashur, R. *Rural health and telecommunications.* Ann Arbor: University of Michigan Press, 1967.

Bass, B. L. *Health care delivery in rural areas.* Chicago: A.M.A., 1972.

Bellin, S. S., & Geiger, H. J. Impact of neighborhood health centers on patient care. *Medical Care*, 1972, *10*, 224.

Bendixen, H. H. Cost of intensive care. In J. Bunker, *Costs, risks, and benefits of surgery.* New York: Oxford University Press, 1977.

Berkonovic, E., & Marcus, A. C. Satisfaction with health services. *Medical Care*, 1976, *14*, 873.

Berkschieder, J. Use of self as the essence of clinical supervision. *Nur. Clin. N.A.*, 1971, *270*, 16.

Blair, W. C., Andersen, M. C., & McNamara, M. J. Comparison of diagnostic costs for hospitalized and ambulatory hypertensive patients. *Inquiry*, 1981, *18*, 37.

Bloom, B. S., Osler, L., & Petersen, M. D. End results, costs and productivity of coronary care units. *New England Journal of Medicine*, 1973, *288*, 11.

Bloom, B. S., & Petersen, O. L. ICU beds in Massachusetts. *New England Journal of Medicine*, 1974, *290*, 1171.

Blumenthal, D. S., McNeal-Steele, M. S., Bullard, L. L., Satcher, D., & Satcher, D. Introducing preclinical students to clinical care. *Journal of Medical Education*, 1983, *58*, 179.

Bognani, S., & Phillips, K. Reducing hospital use in Iowa. *Inquiry*, 1982, *19*, 336.

Bohr, J. M. *Studies on the relationship of elective surgery scheduling to overall hospital occupancy.* Center for Hospital Management, Chicago: A.H.A., 1980.

Bombadier, C., Fuchs, V. R., Lillard, L. A., & Warner, K. E. Socioeconomic factors affecting hospital utilization of surgical operations. *New England Journal of Medicine* 1977, *297*, 699.

Boyle, M. H., Torrance, G. W., Sinclair, J. C., & Harwood, S. P. Economic evaluation of neonatal intensive care units. *New England Journal of Medicine*, 1983, *308*, 1330.

Brand, D. A., Frazier, W. H., Kohlhepp, W. C., Shea, K. M., et al. Protocol for selective patients with injured extremities. *New England Journal of Medicine*, 1982, *306*, 333.

Brickner, P. W. *Home health care for the aged.* Norwalk, CT: Appleton-Century-Crofts, 1978.

Brook, R. H., & Stevenson, R. L. Effectiveness of patient care in emergency rooms. *New England Journal of Medicine,* 1970, *283,* 904.

Brook, R. H., & Appel, F. A. Quality of care assessment. In Kettrie, *Medicine, law and public policy.* New York: A.M.S., 1975.

Brown, J. H. U. *Telecommunications for health care.* Boca Raton: CRC Press, 1982.

Brown, J. H. U. *Politics and health care.* Cambridge, Ma: Ballinger, 1979.

Budetti, P. *Cost effectiveness of neonatal intensive care.* O.T.A., Congress of the United States, Washington, D.C., 1981.

Bunker, J. H. *Costs, risks and benefits of surgery.* New York: Oxford University Press, 1977.

Bunker, J. H., Hinkley, D., & McDermott, W. Surgical innovation and its evaluation. *Science,* 1978, *200,* 937.

Caldwell, K. S., & Brayton, D. Use of TV and film in continuing education. *Journal of Biocommunication,* 1974, *1,* 7.

Campion, E. W. Why acute care hospitals must undertake long term care. *New England Journal of Medicine,* 1983, *308,* 71.

Carels, E. J. *The physician and cost control.* New York: Cambridge University Press, 1980.

Carey, J. *Implementing interactive telecommunications projects.* Alternative Media Center, New York University, 1978.

Caternicchio, R. P., & Davies, R. H. Developing a client focussed allocation of inpatient nursing use. *Sociology and Scientific Medicine,* 1983, *17,* 259.

Chassin, M. R. Costs and outcomes of intensive care. *Medical Care,* 1982, *20,* 161.

Chyba, M. M. *Utilization of hospital emergency and outpatient departments.* National Center for Health Statistics Report #2, Feb. 1983.

Cochrane, A. L. *Effectiveness and efficiency.* National Program Health Technology, London, 1973.

Cohen, A. B., & Cohades, D. R. Certificate of need and low cost medical technology. *Milbank Memorial Fund Quarterly,* 1982, *60,* 307.

Cohen, J. H. A computer based system for detection and prevention of drug reactions. *Drug Information Journal,* 1972, *6,* 81.

Cohen, K. P. *Hospice.* Germantown, Md.: Aspen Press, 1979.

Cole, P. Effective hysterectomy. *New England Journal of Medicine,* 1976, *295,* 264.

Collen, D. J. Survival, hospital charges, and followup in critically ill patients. *New England Journal of Medicine*, 1976, *294*, 983.

*Complex puzzle of rising health care costs.* Council on Wage and Price Administration, Washington, D.C., 1976.

Connelly, D. P., Benson, E. S., Burke, M. D., & Fenderson, D. *Clinical decisions and laboratory use.* University of Minnesota, Minneapolis, 1982.

Connor, R. A. Case based payment systems. *Hospital and Health Service Administration*, 1982, *27*, 39.

Conroth, D. W., Dunn, E. V., Bloom, W. G., & Tranquada, B. Clinical evaluation of four telecommunication systems. *Behavioral Science*, 1979, *22*, 12.

Crile, G., Jr. How to keep down risks and costs of surgery. *Inquiry*, 1981, *18*, 99.

Cromwell, J., & Kanak, J. R. Effect of prospective reimbursement programs on hospital adoption of service sharing. *Health Care Financing Administration H.C.F.R.*, 1982, *4*, 67.

Cromwell, J., & Mitchell, J.B. High income Medicaid practices. *Inquiry*, 1981, *18*, 18.

Cummings, K. M., Frisof, K. B., Long, M. J., & Hrynkiewick, G. Effect of price information on physicians tests ordering behavior. *Medical Care*, 1982, *20*, 293.

Cutler, S. J., Myers, M. H., & Green, S. B. Trends in survival rates of patients with cancer. *New England Journal of Medicine*, 1975, *293*, 122.

Cypress, B. K. *Drug utilization in office visits to primary physicians.* N.C.H.R. Report #86, Oct. 1982.

Cypress, B. K. *Drug utilization in general and family practice by characteristics of physicians and office visits.* N.C.H.S. Report #86, March 1983.

Daniels, M., & Schroeder, S. A. Variations among physicians in the use of laboratory tests. *Medical Care*, 1977, *15*, 482.

Davis, K. Increased numbers of MDs. *John Hopkins Hospital Journal*, 1982, *150*, 55.

Davis, K. Relationships of risks to costs. *Applied Economics*, 1971, *4*, 115.

Davis, M. S. Variations in patients compliance with physicians orders. *Journal of Medical Education*, 1966, *41*, 11.

Dicker, M. *Health care coverage and insurance coverage.* National Center for Health Statistics N.C.H.S. Report #3, May, 1983.

Dixon, R. H. & Laszlo, J. Utilization of clinical chemistry by housestaff. *Archives of Internal Medicine*, 1974, *134*, 1064.

Doerman, A., McArthur, D., & Walcot, P. *Extending the capabilities of physician extenders in rural areas.* McLean, Va.: Mitre Corp., 1975.

Donabedian, A. Quality of medical care. *Science*, 1978, *200*, 856.

*Drugs most frequently used in office practice.* N.C.H.S., May 1982, Washington, D.C.

Dutton, D. B. Patterns of ambulatory care. *Medical Care*, 1979, *17*, 221.

Dyck, F. G., Murphy, F. A., Murphy, J. K., et al. Effect of surveillance on the number of hysterectomies in the province of Saskatchewan. *New England Journal of Medicine*, 1977, *296*, 1328.

Eastbaugh, J. M. Teaching cost effectiveness to medical students. *Inquiry* 1981, *18*, 28.

Eichna, L. W. A medical school curriculum for the 1980s. *New England Journal of Medicine*, 1983, *308*, 19.

Eisenberg, J. M. An educational program to modify lab use by house staff. *Journal of Medical Education*, 1977, *52*, 578.

Eisenberg, J. M., & Kosoff, A. J. Physicians responsibility for the costs of unnecessary services. *New England Journal of Medicine*, 1978, *299*, 76.

Ekwo, E., McDaniels, E., Oliver, D., & Fethke, C. The PA in rural physician practice. *Medical Care*, 1979, *17*, 787.

Elliot, W. B., Strand, H. M., Myers, F. H., et al. Hospital payment capitation project. *Inquiry*, 1983, *20*, 114.

Elnicki, R. A. Substitution of outpatient for inpatient care. *Inquiry*, 1976, *13*, 245.

Enthoven, A. C. Cutting costs without cutting quality. *New England Journal of Medicine*, 1978, *298*, 1229.

Enthoven, A. C. *A health plan.* Reading, Ma.: Addison Wesley, 1980.

Ertel, P. Y., & Aldridge, M. G. *Medical peer reveiw.* St. Louis, Mo.: C. V. Mosby, 1977.

Evans, R. W. Health care technology as the inevitability of resource allocation and rationing decisions. *J.A.M.A.*, 1983, *249*, 2208.

Falter, M. D., & Pinchoff, D. M. Acceptance of the nurse practitioner. *Inquiry*, 1976, *13*, 263.

Feldstein, M. S. *Rising costs of hospital care.* Washington, D.C.: Technical Information Research Services, 1977.

Fetter, R. B., Shin, Y., Freeman, J. L., Averill, R. F., & Thompson, J. D. Case mix definition of DRG. *Medical Care Supplement* (Vol. 18), 1980.

Field, W. G. *Systems in medical care.* Cambridge, Ma.: M.I.T. Press, 1970.

Finkler, S. A. Cost effectiveness of regionalization. *Health Services Research*, 1981, *16*, 327.

Fletcher, R. H., O'Malley, M. S., Earp, J. A., et al. Patient priorties for medical care. *Medical Care*, 1983, *21*, 234.

Freeborn, D. J., Baer, D., & Greenlick, M. R. Determination of medical care utilization. *American Journal of Public Health*, 1972, *62*, 846.

Freeland, M. S., & Schendlet, C. S. National health expenditures growth in the 1980s. *H.C.F.R.*, 1983, *4*, 1.

Fuchs, V. R. *Who shall live?* New York: Basic Books, 1974.

Garrell, M. Organization of a teaching nursing home. *Journal of Medical Education*, 1982, *59*, 482.

Gevarter, W. Expert systems. *I.E.E.E. Spectrum*, 1983, *20*, 39.

Gibson, L. E. Use of water vapor in the treatment of lower respiratory disease. *American Journal Respiratory Disease*, 1974, *110*, Part 2.

Gibson, R. M., & Waldo, D. R. National health expenditures. *H.C.F.R.*, 1982, *4*, 1.

Gilbert, F. L., & Sachs, R. R. Comparisons of health appraisals by nurses and physicians. *Public Health Reports*, 1970, *85*, 1042.

Gilbert, J. P., McPeek, B., & Mosteller, F. Statistics, ethics, and surgery. *Science*, 1977, *198*, 684.

Ginzburg, E., Brann, E. Heistand, D., & Ostov, M. The expanding physician supply. *Milbank Memorial Fund Quarterly*, 1981, *59*, 508.

Ginzburg, E. Procompetition in health care. *Milbank Memorial Fund Quarterly*, 1982, *60*, 386.

Ginzburg, E., & Brann, E. How the medical student views his profession and its future. *Inquiry*, 1980, *17*, 195.

Glen, J. K., & Goldman, J. Strategies for productivity with physician extenders. *Western Journal of Medicine*, 1976, *124*, 249.

Gray, B. *The new health care for profit*. Washington, D.C.: National Academy Press, 1983.

Griner, P. F., & Liptzin, B. Use of the laboratory in a teaching hospital. *Internal Medicine*, 1971, *75*, 157.

Griner, P. F. Treatment of pulmonary edema. *Annual of Internal Medicine*, 1972, *77*, 50.

Griner, P. F. Use of the laboratory in a teaching hospital. *Annual of Internal Medicine*, 1977, *90*, 243.

Harris, D. M. Elaboration of the relationship between general hospital bed supply and utilization. *Journal of Health and Sociological Behavior*, 1975, *16*, 163.

Hauck, W. W., Jr., Bloom, B. S., McPherson, C. K., Nickerson, R. J., et al. Surgeons in the U.S. *J.A.M.A.*,1976, *236*, 1864.

Haverkamp, A., Orleans, M., Langendorfer, S., McFee, J., et al. A controlled trial of fetal monitoring. *American Journal of Obstetrical Gynecology*, 1979, *134*, 399.

Health care financing statistics, 1983, *H.C.F.R. 4*, 115.

Heller, J. A. Unusual aspects of injury in children. *Bibliography on EMS*, DHHS. Washington, D.C., 1976.

Hellinger, F. J. Controlling costs by adjusting payment for medical technologies. *Inquiry*, 1982, *19*, 34.

Herman, C. H., & Rodowska, C. A. Communicating drug information to physicians. *Journal of Medical Education* 1976, *51*, 189.

Herman, C. H., & Rodowska, C. A. Communicating about drugs. *Drug Int. J.* Jan. 1976, p. 20.

Hershey, J. C., & Kroop, D. H. Reappraisal of the productivity potential of physicians assistants. *Medical Care*, 1979, *17*, 592.

Holmes, G. A., Livingston, G., Bassett, R. E., & Mills, E. Nurse clinician productivity. *Health Service Resident,* 1977, *12*, 269.

Homer, C. G. Some pitfalls in creating competition between HMOs and fee for service care. *Journal of Health Public Policy and Law*, 1982, 7, 686.

House Committee on Interstate and Foreign Affairs. *Cost and quality in health care.* Congress of the U.S., Washington, D.C., 1976.

Ingrim, W. B., Hokanson, J. A., Gurngy, B. G., Doutre, W. H., et al. Physician noncompliance with prescription writing requirements. *American Journal of Hospital Pharmacy*, 1983, *40*, 414.

*J.A.M.A. Index issue.* J.A.M.A., Dec. 1982.

Jewesson, P. J., Ho, R., Jang, Q., Watts, G., & Chow, A. W. Auditing antibiotic use in a teaching hospital. *Canadian Medical Association Journal*, 1983, *128*, 1075.

Joffe, J. & Schmidt, T. Effect of task requirements on physician productivity. *Public Health Reports*, 1977, *92*, 147.

Kaluzny, A. D. Innovation in health services. *Health Services Research*, Summer 1974.

Kaluzny, A. D., Veney, J. E., & Gentry, J. T. Predicting two types of hospital innovation. *Health and Hospital Service Administration*, 1976, *21*, 24.

Kessner, D. M., Snow, C. K., & Singer, J. *Assessment of medical care for children.* Washington, D.C.: Institute of Medicine, 1974.

Kirkman, R. Personal Communication.

Klaw, S.. The great American medicine show. New York: Viking Press, 1975.

Knaus, W. A., Wagner, D. P., Draper, E. A., Lawrence, R. E., & Zimmerman, J. F. The range of intensive care. *J.A.M.A.*, 1981, *246*, 2711.

Knowles, J. Doing better and feeling worse. *Daedalus*, Winter, 1977.

Kolata, G. B. Withholding medical treatment. *Science*, 1979, *205*, 882.

Kolata, G. B. Dialysis after a decade. *Science*, 1980, *208*, 473.

Kolata, G. B. Heart transplant—To pay or not to pay. *Science*, 1980, *209*, 570.

Kolata, G. B. Liver transplants endorsed. *Science*, 1983, *221*, 140.

Korenbrot, C., Flood, A. B., Higgins, M., Roos, N., & Bunker J. P. Elective hysterectomy. O.T.A., Congress of the U.S. Washington, 1981.

Kramer, C. *The negligent doctor.* New York: Crown Press, 1978.

Kripne, D. F. Why we need a tax on sleeping pills. *Southern Medical Journal*, 1983, *76*, 632.

Lanin, J. H. They're replacing doctors with nurse practitioners. *Medical Economics*, Jan. 10, 1977, p. 1.

Laurie, R. Operating on children as day cases. *Lancet*, 1964, *20*, 1289.

Law, S., & Polan, S. *Pain and profit.* New York: Harper & Row, 1978.

Lawson, D. H. & Jick, H. Drug prescribing in hospitals. *American Journal of Public Health*, 1976, *66*, 644.

Lee, R. H., & Hedley, J. Physicians fees and the public medical care program. *Health Services Research*, 1981, *16*, 186.

LeRoy, L., & Solkowitz, S. Cost and effectiveness of nurse practitioners. In: *Cost effectiveness of medical technology.* O.T.A., Congress of the U.S., July 1981.

Levit, R. R. Personal health care expenditures. *H.C.F.R.*, 1982, *4*, 1.

Libshitz, H. J. Mammography screening for breast cancer. *Proceedings of the National Cancer Institute*, 1978, *239*, 486.

Lion, J., & Altman, S. Case mix differences between outpatient departments and private practice. *H.C.F.R.*, 1982, *4*, 89.

Logsdon, D. H., Rosen, M. A, & Demoss, M. M. INSURE—A project of life cycle preventive health services. *Inquiry*, 1983, *20*, 121.

Long, M. J., Cummings, K. M., & Frisof, K. B. Role of perceived price in physician demand for diagnostic tests. *Medical Care*, 1983, *21*, 243.

Lubitz, J., & Deacon, R. Rise in the incidence of hospitalization for the aged. *H.C.F.R.*, 1982, *3*, 21.

Luft, H. S., Bunker, J. P., & Enthoven, A. C. Should operations be regionalized. *New England Journal of Medicine*, 1979, *301*, 1364.

McCook, T. A., Ravin, C. E., & Price, R. P. Abdominal radiography in the emergency department. *Annual of Emergency Medicine*, 1982, *11*, 23.

McGee, R. R. Who really cares about medical costs. *Medical Economics*, Feb. 7, 1981, p. 36.

McKibben, R. C. Cost effectiveness of physicians assistants. *Physicians Assistants Journal*, 1978, *8*, 110.

McLachlan, G. *A question of quality.* London: Oxford University Press, 1976.

McLachlan, G., Stocking, B., & Shegog, R. F. H. *Patterns for uncertainty.* London: Oxford University Press, 1979.

McLaughlin, H. Z. *EMS Conference report.* Jacksonville, EMS, 1975.

McNiel, B. J., Keller, E., & Adelstein, S. J. Primer of elements in decision making. *New England Journal of Medicine*, 1975, *293*, 211.

MacStravic, R. E. Admission scheduling and capacity pooling. *Inquiry*, 1981, *18*, 345.

Making your practice malpractice proof (Editorial). *Medical Economics*, July, 1975, p. 4.

Maloney, T., & Rogers, D. Medical technology. *New England Journal of Medicine*, 1979, *301*, 1413.

Maloney, L. New understanding about death. *U.S. News and World Report*, July 11, 1983, p. 69.

Marshal, C. L. & Wallerstein, F. *To establish a directional communication system.* DHHS, Washington, D.C. 1973.

Martin, S. P., Donaldson, M. C., London, C. D., Peterson, O. L., & Colton, T. Inputs into coronary care during 30 years. *Annual of Internal Medicine*, 1974, *81*, 289.

Martz, E. W., & Ptakowski, R. Educational costs to hospitalized patients. *Journal of Medical Education*, 1978, *53*, 383.

Medical research, statistics, and ethics. (Symposium). *Science*, 1977, *198*, 677.

Meskewskas, J. A., Benson, J. A., & Hopkins, E. Performance of FMGs on examination by American Board of Internal Medicine. *New England Journal of Medicine*, 1977, *297*, 808.

Mitchell, J. B., & Cromwell, J. Medicaid mills—Fact or fiction. *H.C.F.R.*, Summer 1980.

Mitchell, J. B., & Cromwell, J. Large Medicaid practices and Medicaid bills. *J.A.M.A.*, 1980, *244*, 2433.

Mitchell, J. B., & Cromwell, J. Impact on all or nothing assignment with Medicare. *H.C.F.R.*, 1983, *4*, 59.

Moore, F. D., & Long, S. M. Board Certified Physicians in the U.S. *New England Journal of Medicine*, 1981, *304*, 1079.

Morehead, M. A. *Quality hospital care.* New York: Columbia University Press, 1964.

Morrisey, M. A., & Ashley, C. S. An empirical analysis of HMO market shares. *Inquiry*, 1982, *19*, 136.

Moses, L. E., & Mosteller, F., Jr. *J.A.M.A.*, 1968, *203*, 422.

Moss, F. M., McNichol, M. W., McSwiggen, D. A., & Miller, D. Survey of antibiotic prescribing in a general hospital. *Lancet*, 1981, *2*, 461.

Murphy, M. L., Hultgren, H. N., Detre, K., Thomsen, J., & Tokaro, T. Treatment of chronic stable angina. *New England Journal of Medicine*, 1977, *297*, 621.

Murphy, R. L. H. Microwave transmission of chest x-ray. *American Journal of Respiratory Diseases*, 1970, *102*, 771.

Muskin, L. P., & Dunlap, D. V. *Health—What is it worth?* New York: Pergamon Press, 1979.

Myers, L. P., & Schroeder, S. A. Physicians use of services for the hospitalized patient. *Milbank Memorial Fund Quarterly*, 1981, *59*, 481.

Neuhauser, D., & Lewicki, L. What we gain from a sixth stool guaiac. *New England Journal of Medicine*, 1978, *293*, 266.

Newhouse, J. *The demand for medical services.* Santa Monica, Ca.: Rand Corp, 1980.

Oatman, E. F. *Medical care in the U.S.* New York: H. W. Wilson Co., 1978.

Orient, J. M., Kettel, L. J., Sox, H. C., Jr., Sox, C. H., et al. Effect of treatment algorithms on quality of patient care. *Medical Care*, 1983, *21*, 157.

Othensmeger, D. J., & Smith, H. L. Opportunities for established group practices. *New England Journal of Medicine*, 1982, *306*, 74.

Owen, A. How much is board certification worth? *Medical Economics*, Jan 10, 1983, p. 58.

Owen, A. Where the primary care squeeze is hurting. *Medical Economics*, June 19, 1983, p. 104.

Paris, M. Cost and quality control of laboratory services. *Medical Care*, 1976, *14*, 777.

Paroles, J. Effects of health services on adult mortality. In: *Costs of health care.* Fogarty International Center, DHHS, Washington, D.C., 1976.

Pascarelli, E. F. *Hospital based ambulatory care.* Norwalk, Ct.: Appleton-Century-Croft, 1982.

Patrick, J. D., Doris, P. E., Mills, M. L., Friedman, J., & Johnson, C. Lumbar spine x-rays. *Annual of Emergency Medicine*, 1983, *12*, 84.

Pettigrew, L. C. *The patient as client.* Master's thesis, University of Texas, Houston, 1981.

Rafferty, J. *Health manpower and productivity.* Lexington, Ma.: Lexington Books, 1974.

Raimtoola, S. H., Nemby, D., Grumkemeier, G., Tepley, J., et al. Ten year survival after coronary bypass surgery. *New England Journal of Medicine*, 1983, *308*, 676.

Rastuccia, J. D., & Murphy, D. V. Estimating hospital costs by DRG. *Inquiry*, 1980, *17*, 155.

Reich, J. J. *Telecommunications.* Washington University, St. Louis, 1974.

Retting, R. A. Politics of health cost containment. *Bulletin of N.Y. Academy of Medicine*, 1980, *56*, 115.

Retting, R. A. *Formal analysis, policy formulation, and end stage renal disease.* O.T.A., Congress of the U.S., Washington, D.C., April 1981.

Robinson, G. C., & Clark, H. F. *Hospital care of children.* New York: Oxford University Press, 1980.

Roemer, M. I. More data on surgical deaths related to the 1976 physician slowdown. *Social Science and Medicine*, 1981, *15*, 99.

Roos, N. P., & Roos, L. L. High and low surgical rates. *American Journal of Public Health*, 1981, *71*, 591.

Roos, L. L. Supply, workload & utilization. *American Journal of Public Health*, 1983, *73*, 414.

Ross, S. A. The clinical nurse practitioner. *Bulletin of N.Y. Academy of Medicine*, 1977, *49*, 393.

Salawey, V. K. Managing variability in demand. *H.C.F.R.*, 1982, 7, 37.

Sawyer, T. Pharmaceutical reimbursement and drug cost control. *Inquiry*, 1983, *20*, 76.

Schachter, K., & Neuhouse, D. *Surgery for breast cancer.* O.T.A., Congress of the U.S., Washington, D.C., 1981.

Scheffler, R. M., & Delaney, M. *Assessing selected respiratory therapy modulities.* O.T.A., Congress of the U.S., Washington, D.C., 1981.

Schneeswiss, R. Diagnostic Clusters. *Medical Care*, 1983, *21*, 105.

Schoenbaum, S. C., Hyde, J. N., Bartoshevsky, L., & Crampton, K. Cost benefit of rubella vaccination policy. *New England Journal of Medicine* 1976, *294*, 306.

Schroeder, S. A., & O'Leary, D. S. Differences in laboratory use and the length of stay in university and community hospitals. *Journal of Medical Education*, 1977, *52*, 418.

Scitovsky, A. A., & McCall, N. *Changes in the costs of treatment*. DHEW 77-3161 Washington, D.C., 1976.

Scott, W. R., Forrest, W. H., & Brown, B. W., Jr. *Organizational research in hospitals*. Blue Cross Association, Chicago, 1976.

Showstock, J. A., & Schroeder, S. A. *Cost effectiveness of upper GI endoscopy*. O.T.A., Congress of the U.S., Washington, D.C., 1981.

Slack, W. V., & VanCura, L. J. Patient reactions to computer based interviews. *Computers in Biomedical Research*, 1968, *1*, 527.

Smith, D. B., & Kaluzny, A. D. *The white labyrinth*. Berkeley, Ca.: McCutcheon Publishing, 1975.

Smith, F. E., Trivax, G., Zuehlke, D. A., Lowingen, P., & Noheim, T. L. Health information during a week of TV. *New England Journal of Medicine*, 1972, *288*, 516.

Solon, J. A., & Greenwalt, L. F. Physicians participating in nursing homes. *Medical Care*, 1974, *12*, 486.

Spencer, D. L., & D'Elia, G. Effect of regional medical education on physician distribution. *Journal of Medical Education*, 1983, *58*, 309.

Spiegel, A. D., & Burkhart, B. H. *Curing and caring*. New York: S.P. Medical Science Books, 1980.

Spiegel, J. S., Rubenstein, L. V., Scott, B., & Brooks, R. H. Who is the primary physician? *New England Journal of Medicine*, 1983, *308*, 1208.

Stump, I. G. Are diagnostic tests repeated unnecessarily? *Canadian Medical Association Journal*, 1983, *128*, 1185.

Sussman, E. J., Eisenberg, J. M., & Williams, S. V. Diagnostic services Review. *H.C.F.R.*, 1981, *6*, 65.

Tancredi, L. R., & Barondess, J. A. Problems of defensive medicine. *Science*, 1978, *200*, 879.

Tatchell, M. Measuring hospital output. *Social Science Medicine*, 1983, *17*, 87.

Weemstein, M. C. *Cost effectiveness of medical technology*. O.T.A., Congress of the U.S., Washington, D.C., 1981.

Weissant, W. F., Wan, T. T. H., Livieratos, B. B., & Pelligrino, J. Cost effectiveness of home services for the chronically ill. *Inquiry*, 1980, *17*, 230.

Wennberg, J. E., & Gittleson, A. Small area variations in health care delivery. *Scientific American* 1982, *246*, 120.

Wheeler, M. F., Wilson, L. D., & Wood, R. H. Algorithms directed care by non-physician practitioners in a pediatric population. *Medical Care*, 1983, *21*, 138.

Williams, K. N., & Brook, R. H. *Foreign medical graduates and their effect on quality of care*. Santa Monica, Ca.: Rand Corp, 1976.

Williams, S. G., Eisenberg, J. M., Pascale, L. A., & Kitz, D. S. Perceptions about unnecessary diagnostic testing. *Inquiry*, 1982, *19*, 363.

Wolensky, F. D., & Marder, W. D. Organization of medical practice and primary physician income. *American Journal Public Health*, 1983, *73*, 379.

Wong, Mccarron, E. T., & Shaw, S. T., Jr. Ordering lab tests in a teaching hospital. *J.A.M.A.*, 1983, *249*, 3090.

Wood, C. T. Relating hospital charges to use of services. *Harvard Business Review*, 1982, *60*, 123.

Wren, F. R. Neurosurgery in the Carolinas. *Clinical Neurology*, 1975, *22*, 539.

Zeleznick, C., Hojat, M., & Veluski, J. Baccalaureate preparation for medical school. *Journal Medical Education*, 1983, *58*, 58.

# INDEX